And Then

THERE WERE THREE

One Sister's Journey through the Heartbreak of Covid

LYNDA ARMES

Lynda

Library of Congress Control Number: 021911464

ISBN: 978-1-7373660-0-3

First Printing: June 2021

Published by RA Estates, Inc.
Folsom, CA 95630

Cover photos by Kate Newman Farlee

Dedication

To the memory of my sister, who got it right the first time. Her smile and laughter will never be forgotten. Her total love of life and the joy she brought to most every occasion were her gift, as well as her legacy. Amazing only begins to describe her.

To my husband, Sam, and my grandson, Christian for all they have had to endure and their unconditional love.

To all those who suffered a loss from Covid as well as my "soul" survivors.

Table of Contents

Chapter 1 The Beginning

It was the best of times, it was the worst of times…
~ Charles Dickens

Indeed, it was supposed to be the best of times. Still, life's fickle finger of fate came sneaking up and tapped me on the shoulder. My story begins just six months before January 2020, a year that changed the lives of many of us forever.

Relaxing at the pub table in the dining area off the kitchen, and sharing a glass of my favorite Cabernet Sauvignon with my only sister, Sandy, while my sister-in-law, Barbara, sipped on her Stella Artois, we could hardly contain our excitement. We had recently learned of the upcoming wedding of my granddaughter Megan and her long-time beau, Rico. The wedding was to be in Orlando, Florida, in the springtime. A destination wedding; what fun!

The "boys" were in the family room watching

baseball. My husband, Sam, was fooling with the remote temperature/timer for the Traeger grill. Glen, my brother, was making sure everyone was comfortable and my brother-in-law Jim had his little cooler of beer next to the recliner. I am not a beer aficionado, and since there are way too many choices these days, I ask beer drinkers to bring their own. Christian, our grandson, who at the age of nine is an "old soul" was there too, feeling every bit a part of the group.

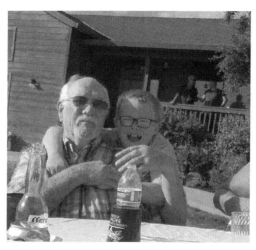

Sibling Sunday had been a regular monthly food fest for a couple of years. My love for cooking and my desire to spend time with my brothers and sister was important to me. Sandy's cooking fame was limited to Dump Cakes, KFC, Stouffer's Lasagna, and all things frozen, so she volunteered to bring snacks or dessert. Glen supplied something yummy, so there was always an abundance of food and laughter.

The wedding was only one topic of conversation.

As the weeks rolled from summer to fall, cheering on New England, Dallas, and the Raiders would be a Sunday staple. Other subjects such as upcoming hot rod weekends, RV traveling, and family matters were also on the agenda. Sandy was going to be a great-grandmother in February of 2020. One spoiled baby girl on its way.

Unfortunately, my brother Rick, and his wife, Kate, couldn't be with us. They lived quite a distance, and Kate was studying hard for a test that might land her a promotion so time was a precious commodity.

We were discussing plans for all of us to travel together to the wedding and vacation afterward. This would be the first time since childhood that all of us, including our spouses, would be spending any extended time in the same house. I know I felt a little bit of trepidation, and I am sure the others did too.

My brother, Glen was the first to be born into our family. Two and a half years later, Sandy was born. There was a five and a half-year gap before I popped in and another five and a half years for our brother Rick to round out the four of us. We were siblings, but all very different. What an adventure we were about to have!

First, we had to decide when we would leave. Do we plan a vacation for all of us before the wedding, after the wedding, or a bit of both? How much time do we want to spend? Even though only two of us were still employed, there were other considerations, like our beloved furry families. Then, of course, what do we want to experience? What is going on in Orlando other than the wedding? When you are flying across the country you want to make every minute count. I reminded the girls how I had experienced flight delays that took us almost two days longer to get to Megan's college graduation in Bowling Green, Ohio, from Sacramento that included an unplanned overnight in Denver, so I did not want to take any chances. Arriving three days before the wedding seemed perfect.

Christian was the ring bearer for the wedding, and Sam and I being the grandparents of the bride, needed to be at the rehearsal on Friday afternoon. Christian felt so important.

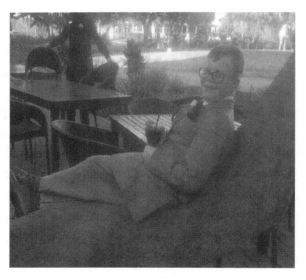

He loved his "Nonnie," a name he gave Megan when they first met. He was two at the time. They would cuddle up and watch Disney movies, especially *CARS*. Rico was also great with Christian and had been so good to him whenever they were visiting from

Florida. They would lay on the playroom floor and put Legos together.

We had Thursday before the wedding designated as a Disney day, and then Friday and Saturday were committed to the wedding. We figured Sunday we would need to relax and we thought it wise to avoid the weekend crowds. We did the math and to squeeze in everything we had planned it needed to be a 10-day trip; departure on the red-eye on March 10 and return on March 21, 2020.

June not only brought sunshine, Sandy's birthday, and summer plans, it also brought news that Sandy's husband, Jim, had an incurable lung disease. The prognosis was a life span of approximately two years, depending on how aggressive the disease chose to be. Of course, the news shook us all badly, but our family is not high on drama or missing a good time, so we began to make plans that were flexible enough to include the possibility that Sandy and Jim might have to cancel.

Sam and I took responsibility for doing all the research and making reservations, as we both were a bit more computer savvy. What was I thinking? We had not done any trip planning for a few years. Keeping Jim in mind, we knew we had to have a ground floor unit if we went with a condo or townhouse or a downstairs bedroom and bath if we rented a house.

It was immediately apparent we were not the only ones needing or desiring such units. Did you know there are entire subdivisions devoted to Disney travelers? Row after row, street after street, filled with townhouses, condos, and four, five, and six-bedroom houses, all within a short distance of all the things Orlando-Kissimmee had to offer.

Two of our kids had made reservations at a development called Windsor Hills, so that is where the housing search began. After an intense two-month search, we decided to reserve two different units. We needed to be flexible. Jim was scheduled to see his doctor in January 2020, and we would know then if they could make the trip. My brother Rick had generously offered to pick up Sandy's and Jim's quarter share of the expenses if they could not go and the travel insurance did not come through.

I booked a three-bedroom condo, as well as a six-bedroom, two-story house with a pool and spa. Since the subdivision had a huge community pool, water park, slides, a large gathering space, an exercise gym, and a small store, we felt set for the ultimate vacation vibe.

Next up was planning our excursions. My brother Rick and I grew up as New York Yankee baseball fans. I was always more interested in sports than "girl" things. I was twelve when the Yankees won the World Series. I was so excited I ran around the block in celebration. Considering we lived in the country, that block was over a mile.

I am such a fan that when my husband and I visited Boston, I dragged him to Fenway Park to see the infamous Red Sox/Yankee rivalry in action. When Rick called and said the Yankees would be in Tampa for spring training while we were in Florida, my brother

Glen and I decided the three of us would go.

Rick's wife Kate researched alligator hydroplane boat rides, and she found one that sounded adventuresome. Of course, we all agreed on that. Airboats are a blast. And no trip to Florida should be without alligator sightings.

I found the Hoop De Doo Review online, a Disney favorite. My kids had seen it and absolutely loved it. It's a rowdy dinner show with live music and the Disney touch. We already knew Epcot, Disney World, Animal Kingdom, Universal Studios, and Hollywood Studios were on the list. The only indecision was whether to try to squeeze in the Kennedy Space Center, Daytona, or a beach day. And we had to visit Disney Springs; the shopping/dining district at Disney World. Would we have time for all these events and be able to relax too?

Good news came in January when the doctor gave the go-ahead for Jim to travel with us. Arrangements were made for an electric wheelchair to be delivered to our rental in Florida for the duration of our trip so Jim could enjoy everything he wanted to do. The beauty of the home was that if you didn't feel like going out with everyone, it was a comfortable place with lots to do.

Eventually, all the reservations for accommodations, airline tickets, wheelchair assistance, excursions, and, of course, a vehicle to carry the seven of us were completed. Rick and Kate were flying in a day later and departing a day before our plans so they were renting another vehicle. We had plenty of room for nine travelers.

Chapter 2 Imperfectly Perfect

For me personally, the two biggest decisions were my dress and my "bags." For much of my adult life I suffered from extreme allergies and somewhere along the way, the bags beneath my eyes began to resemble one of those bug-eyed South American bullfrogs. REALLY! The airlines could have charged me extra baggage fees whenever I flew.

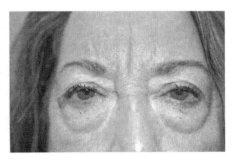

I visited my optometrist in September and she recommended I have my droopy upper lids tightened to improve my sight. I asked her about the possibility of having my lower "droopy" lids done at the same time.

What a great opportunity that would be.

I was determined at last not to take those bags with me. She referred me to a specialist who then referred me to a surgeon. I thought starting the process in September would give me plenty of time. It never occurred to me how popular cosmetic surgery was in California. My surgery did not get scheduled until February. Just six weeks before the wedding and barely in time to be recovered. Little did I know that a few weeks later nobody would notice my "new" eyes covered by a mask.

But of course, this was almost a disaster. My surgeon had failed to schedule the most important part of the surgery; my "bags." Heart palpitations!! Thankfully, the surgery after mine was canceled and she was able to rearrange the schedule. Once that was accomplished, I moved on to finding the "perfect" attire for the grandmother of the bride.

What began as casual perusing on the internet in September, gave way to a full-on assault by my sister, one of my closest friends, Louise, as well as myself by November. I looked at so many dresses, I thought my eyes would actually fall out of their sockets at one point. I was very self-conscious of my appearance: short, knobby-knees, bat wings. I knew a tent would not do, but what else would cover all those flaws?

Then, it happened. Three months after my shopping began and three months before the wedding. It was early December and I saw THE perfect outfit; the color and everything. Elation! I emailed a photo to my "advisors" and everyone agreed it was ME. The search was over, but I had a six to eight-week wait for delivery. I had never seen a pantsuit like this. It was three pieces of soft chiffon. The sleeveless shell had a vertical, tiered hem. The jacket had a cropped bodice in front that flowed in a tiered fashion on the back and sides across the hips, with three-quarter-length sleeves. Truly understated, yet elegant attire for a semi-formal evening wedding. It would cover all of my flaws beautifully. I was measured for a custom fit. I couldn't wait to see it on.

Everything was coming together.

Just before the anticipated arrival, my daughter-in-law had experienced a panicky situation. Kelli had purchased her gown from a Bay area specialty shop. When it finally arrived at the dress shop, a month later than originally scheduled, they sent it on to Kelli. The promised delivery date came and went—no dress. The post office tracking number found it had been shipped to the North Coast town of Eureka, three hundred miles away! Worse yet, they stated it could be caught in a "loop" and had no idea when it might get out of the loop and be delivered. Kelli's sigh of relief when it arrived could be heard globally!

Now I began to get worried and started emailing my dressmaker. I was assured the pantsuit was on its way.

The day I came home from my outpatient eye surgery was the same day my pantsuit arrived. Even though I was in a bit of a drug haze, I could tell this silky item was NOT my pantsuit, but someone's lingerie. OMG…no…utter disbelief. What went wrong? My perfect planning, my perfect pantsuit…and less than six weeks before we leave.

Where is my pantsuit and what have they done with it!

The company I ordered my pantsuit from had no idea what had gone wrong and was absolutely no help in solving the situation. They offered to send a replacement for more money. Are you kidding! My perfect pantsuit, lost. The battle lines were drawn. There were multiple carriers involved and each denied responsibility. I was determined, yes, tenacious, in my search for resolution.

I noticed the courier had delivered from a transfer hub in Southern California, so I called, emailed, and Facebooked until I received another unsatisfactory answer. Then a thought of genius surfaced. I noticed my address label had another label beneath it, as did the return address label. I plugged in my steam iron and steamed away. Yep, it worked! Not easy mind you, but doable. The item I received was to have gone to France. I was getting closer.

With a bit more detective work, I was able to reach a wonderful young woman who worked for the shipping company that originated the shipment. She immediately saw the error. Interestingly enough, the dressmaker had already contacted them. You know, the one who offered to make a new one for more money? That dressmaker had been reimbursed by the shipping company for the lost package. Well, my new best friend at the shipping company contacted the dressmaker and made them aware of the need to reimburse me. Even though I had uncovered the mystery, this took weeks, so it was too late for anything but off-the-rack shopping.

The next weeks could only be described as ugly. Desperately ugly. I could not go out and shop myself because of the eye surgery. I took photos of items I already had in my closet and tried them on. They weren't quite the fresh, light look for a Florida spring wedding. And I had gone up one full size since they were purchased. My closet choices were not going to Florida. Once my daughter-in-law, Kelli, the bride's mom, saw them, I began receiving text messages from her with photos of dresses. Yes, she went shopping. My selfies had definitely spurred her into action, shopping and taking pictures on her phone for my thumbs up or thumbs down. Only one looked promising so home it came.

But I was not sure if this one was IT. The dresses rolled in: Macy's, Nordstrom's, Bloomingdale's. As with many outfits, they often look much better on the hanger or in a picture. By the time I tried them on there was a definite disconnect. I am guessing that at one point I had nearly $2,000.00 in dresses shipped, tried on, and rejected in one week. And then I still had shoes, jewelry, and a handbag to acquire.

But then, just like that, it happened. Isn't it funny how things work out? I was intent on finding a casual lounging outfit for our vacation when I decided to check out the clearance rack at a discount chain store. At the end were a few evening dresses. Hmm. I rarely shopped at this store and I definitely was not looking to buy THE dress here. The sizes were all very large, and then, there it was, the only one in my size. In the wedding's color. On sale. I recognized the dressmaker. Was this too good to be true? Less than three weeks to go. I hurried to the dressing room. Prayerfully, I put it on. Eureka! Still time to get it to the tailor to have alterations made.

Better even than my first choice and hundreds of dollars less expensive. It was a navy-blue, one-piece jumpsuit. One bare shoulder hosted a strap only. The opposite shoulder had an elbow-length sleeve with a sequined overlay that crossed the bodice and went down the opposite side to the bottom hem of the pants. It would hide everything! Well, almost. Only an obsessed "Oma" of the bride would understand.

Finally, I could relax. I ordered silver evening pumps, a handbag, and some costume jewelry to complement the diamond bracelet and earrings I would wear.

Orlando, brace yourself! We're coming.

Chapter 3 A Trip to Remember

In January 2020, I became increasingly aware of a virus that was coming to the USA via China. It was at that time, Dr. Fauci, Director of the National Institute of Allergy and Infectious Diseases, began assuring us that, although it was a serious virus, there was nothing to be concerned about. I had gotten my annual lung infection and Sandy had her perpetually bad-sounding cough. We had plenty of time to get over them.

That was good news. I had a wedding and a grand vacation to prepare for. My siblings were all on board. We joked about how the virus was named after a beer. Yes, the Corona Virus, since renamed Covid-19, was making the news.

Megan flew in from Florida and two of her college roommates flew in from Ohio for her bridal shower and bachelorette party. It was a nice day in January for a brunch overlooking the Sacramento River. I was the designated driver for Sandy, Barb, and myself. One of my gifts to the bride was a cookbook of my mother's, from the 1930s. And yes, there were tears. My mom was dearly missed. We're getting closer to the big day and she would be so excited if she were still here.

As of late February, only 2,008 people in China had died, with 83,000 cases reported worldwide. Not much to worry about, however, I kept Jim top of mind.

With four auto-immune system diseases, plus environmental, as well as food allergies, I accepted the fact that if anyone got it, it would be me. Since very little was actually known about the virus, I continued to concentrate on the list of things I could control. I was to learn much later how small that list could be. Being fearless has its advantages at times.

The thought of getting a bad case of the flu was not pleasant, but I was not missing the wedding on the off chance I would get sick. By late February, there were sixty-eight confirmed cases in the US. Again, nothing alarming, and none of us were concerned about contracting the disease.

I feel it was the fact that it was a virus that kept my concern minimal. My entire life, when I was diagnosed with a virus, there was no prescription, no cure. Rest, plenty of fluids, and Ibuprofen. Easy. It is now February 28, less than two weeks before we are to board for our flight, a total of sixty-four US citizens have died from the virus, but they were elderly. Ironically, not one of my siblings, although we were all "age-qualified" considered ourselves elderly. Our conversations were about the wedding, fun, and more fun. That, and the news that Sandy's grandson was getting married in June. More excitement for our family. There was no talk or concern over the virus amongst us. I had envisioned a full ten days of non-stop Sibling Sunday comradery. Our universal distrust of any news reporting regarding the virus had already begun.

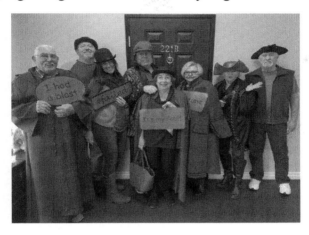

Just two days before we were to leave, Dr. Fauci, in an interview with *60 Minutes,* said that masks were only necessary for those diagnosed with the virus. Others could opt to wear them, however, it only served to make them feel better. Since my pharmacy was out of masks, this was a big relief.

About that same time, Christian heard something about the dangers of flying on planes that caused him to experience some anxiety and concern. What do we do now? One of the many "talking heads" was expounding on international travel. To a nine-year-old that included Florida. Once again, the onslaught of sensationalized reporting was creating an atmosphere of fear as well as mistrust.

Americans seemed to have been shocked out of

their minds amid wealth building, prosperity, and peace. There was now the uncertainty of their future. People became obsessed with finding any news that would return them to that life again. Instead, they were filled with relentless negative suppositions. Fear of the pandemic grew. Conflicting reports surfaced daily. Who would survive? Who was likely to die? Is my family next? Would we ever return to normal?

What happened to who, what, where, when, and how, the basic tenets of any news story? Sadly, it has been replaced by opinion, supposition, could be, possibly, unnamed sources, and snippets of spoken words taken out of context.

On to the final packing. Sandy and I talked a lot about what to take. Since we had a pool and spa at our rental, I decided to finally buy a Miracle Suit. For those who do not know what a miracle suit is, I can tell you firsthand, there is no MIRACLE. The glowing reviews and photos of women looking shapely in their suits caused me to whip out the Mastercard and order a suit of primarily greens and blues that looked perfectly tropical. Besides, it was on sale. I will only say that the most exercise I got on the trip was putting my body into that suit.

Moving on from what to wear, I realized we needed transportation to the airport. Do you have any idea how many suitcases are required for seven people for a ten-day trip? We had not really considered the number of suitcases that would be required. None of the transportation services we contacted could handle the combination of travelers and suitcases in one van.

Thankfully, my good friends Ed and Teri volunteered to pick us up in two vehicles. One more item off the list.

Earlier in March, my BFF since age five phoned from Arizona. She knew my family well. In fact, her younger brother and my brother Rick were also friends since childhood. When I told her of our plans, she questioned whether we should be traveling and asked me to reconsider. She had just canceled a trip to Idaho to celebrate her father's ninety-fifth birthday. She was well aware of my health issues and did not like the prospect of my being exposed to this virus. It was then I reminded her, "Fear not for I am with you" is my firm belief. Being at my granddaughter's wedding and sharing this occasion with the sibs was just too important. We were all in agreement that the small chance of getting the virus was not going to deter us.

Finally, March 10th arrived. My two siblings and their spouses began arriving at my home early in the afternoon. Rick and Kate would follow on a Thursday flight. Sam and I had a habit of packing the day we were leaving. Sandy was a bit unnerved by the fact I was still packing when she arrived. Being late to the airport was not on her schedule!

The fun had begun. Sandy and I laughed when we saw we had both purchased an abundance of wipes, as well as hand sanitizers in multiple sizes. I had two masks. The last two that another local pharmacy had in stock. It was amazing to me that with few people wearing masks, the pharmacies did not seem to have any.

You may well be wondering by now just what in

the world were these siblings thinking? Ranging in age from sixty-eight to seventy-nine, traveling across the country for ten days, and packing in so many activities with a virus beginning to spread. You may have sensed that we are just pretty average people who check things out, calculate the costs, as well as the risks, and go from there. You may have also sensed that as a group, we were a force to be reckoned with…and we were going to Florida. We had travel insurance; paid in advance for our excursions, as well as our accommodations. The news of Covid was not alarming to us at that time. No one among us had any fear or even considered not going.

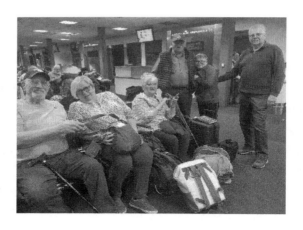

We arrived at the airport early, so we could have dinner there before we boarded. One of the nicest airline transportation employees we encountered on our trip greeted Jim curbside and escorted us through check-in, security, and to the restaurant. Sandy and I began wiping the table, chair surfaces, and silverware.

We thought we were so virus savvy. Our pre-flight dinner at The Iron Horse was excellent. We had time to relax and get into vacation mode.

Once on the plane, we wiped down every seat, headrest, armrest, overhead panel, and window area of all of our seats, and strapped ourselves in. Prepared for takeoff.

Everyone was a bit sleep-deprived upon arrival at Orlando International. Sam and Glen went to take care of getting the seven-passenger rental van. We girls had arranged for private transportation and took a few bags with us, while Jim and Christian waited in the terminal for Sam to return with the van to load the balance of the bags, then meet us at our Florida "home."

The ride from the airport in the pre-dawn light was not that pretty. The shadows and outlines of the foliage were not of palm trees, but dark, almost menacing shapes. Not tropical or exciting. I had been to Orlando four times previously and never noticed. Hopefully, it was just the time of the morning, I thought. It was a bit disappointing and seems to me now that it was a fore-shadowing of what was to come.

Upon entering our two-story, temporary home, the muted grey walls with a playful touch of tangerine welcomed us into our peaceful sanctuary. To the left was the living room furnished with a leather sofa and a love seat. Next to it, was a dining room with a window-shaped opening to the kitchen. It allowed for us to have a quiet space, yet still be connected.

To the right, near the foot of the stairs, was an entry table with a state-of-the-art video monitor above it showing restaurants, the clubhouse, and a variety of opportunities to interact and make reservations. Technology was evident throughout the home. Upstairs there were two master suites, three more large bedrooms, and a large bath.

Downstairs had cool tile flooring and the remainder was the well-appointed kitchen with a breakfast bar, a small eating area family room combo, and an additional bedroom, bath, and laundry area.

The sliding glass door off the eating area leading to a screened-in patio with a large heated (optional) pool and spa, also had a unique safety feature. You had to push a button BEFORE opening the slider both to go out and come back in or a shrieking alarm went off. Can you say extremely annoying!!

The patio area had a BBQ, a large dining table with chairs, and several loungers. The garage had been converted into a game room with air hockey, a jukebox, pool table, and ping pong, and completed the 3000-sq. ft. plus home.

After a few hours of sleep/rest, it was off to fill the pantry and refrigerator. Just down the street was the biggest Walmart I have ever seen. We loaded up with cleaning supplies, food, and beverages, and settled in. Barbara had come along, but we soon lost her to the lure of shopping. After all, this was the largest Walmart ever, I am sure. Before we knew it, she had gone exploring. When all the shopping was done and the ice cream was melting, we still hadn't found her. I told you this was a big store, right? After being told the store's intercom system had been down for a couple of weeks and there were no "lost shopper" paging calls going out, we fanned out row by row and finally found her, or she had found us. She had already begun "souvenir" gathering. She LOVES shopping!

We all got up Thursday morning to head for Animal Kingdom. We picked up one of our grandsons and met up with other family members already there. The vacation had officially begun.

Animal Kingdom is THE most popular park, and I was so excited to share it with my siblings. The Safari was a top Orlando attraction. Long lines awaited the opportunity to board a "safari vehicle" and be driven through the natural habit where animals roamed freely. It never occurred to me they would not enjoy it, but Glen and Sandy thought it was nothing more than visiting a zoo.

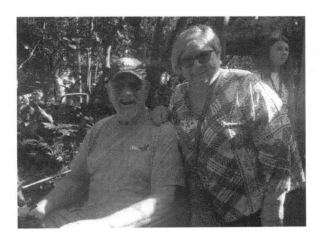

I guess my description of the personal experience I had had two years previously did not quite meet their expectations. I felt bad that they were disappointed. I had tried to make this vacation a dream vacation for everyone. Not a good start, but I would make it up somehow. We had plenty of adventures planned.

As we returned to our Florida home, the news of the virus was beginning to sound ominous. We were all pretty skeptical by now. We were in Florida and not witnessing anything that was being reported. Ignoring the drama of the evening news, we relaxed, kicked back, and began reviewing plans for the next day. Tomorrow was the wedding rehearsal and then THE wedding.

Rick and Kate were flying in that evening late, so being fun-loving siblings, we thought it would be hysterical to short-sheet their bed. You can imagine our disappointment the next morning when they got up and had to be told what we had done. Apparently, they were too tired to notice. So far nothing was going as expected.

Each of us began receiving concerned texts from family and friends in California, as well as those who were in Florida for the wedding. We were all getting different questions and hearing different stories. Still not much was definitive. Most of the news was speculation and pondering. We knew one thing for sure. We were going to a wedding. The ceremony, as well as the reception, were being held at the Historic Dubsdread Ballroom in Orlando.

It was the first time I was to meet the groom's family. They reside in Maywood, New Jersey so we had only been Facebook friends, as well as having had calls and messages for almost a year. Susan was as anxious as I was to finally meet. Very gracious and loving. We hugged immediately. It was so special and reflective of how the entire Pasamba family is.

At the rehearsal dinner, there were thirty-five people all chatting excitedly about the wedding and sharing the latest on what was happening in Florida, and, more specifically, the Orlando area because of the virus. No one was concerned or expressing anxiety.

Things began to change rapidly. It was that very evening, the Friday before the wedding that the decision to close Disney World and Universal Studios came. On only our third day of "dream vacation." We were all shocked. Sunday, following the wedding, would be the last day for any amusement parks to be open. Disney Springs, which is the entertainment and shopping district, was to remain open, but the park itself would be temporarily closed. At least we would have some part of the Disney experience to share.

Everyone began making plans for Sunday and what they wanted to do for the only amusement park day we would have. We also planned all the logistics for everyone to get to the wedding venue on Saturday evening; the reason we all came to Florida, Megan and Rico's wedding!

The two had met while attending Disney College. Megan had been a "Disney Girl" from an early age. She had a collection of just about every Disney movie ever released and visiting the Magic Kingdom was always on her list of things to do. While attending college in Ohio, she applied for a semester at Disney College and was accepted. Being a California girl, she had visited Disneyland in Anaheim many times, but she had only been to Disney World once.

You can imagine the excitement when she got her acceptance letter that she was going to Disney College. She would get college credit for the entire semester doing something she'd dreamed about. Was this around when you were attending college? While there, she would work for the Disney Corporation, as well as take educational courses. Oh, did I mention they had a lot of fun, also? She was attending Bowling Green University in Ohio and Rico, who was from New Jersey, attended college in New York. So it was that these two college kids came to meet and fall in love.

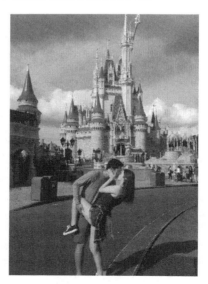

They both got their first jobs with the Disney Corporation after college graduation. Rico graduated a year ahead of Meg, so he was settled in Orlando and waiting for her when she said goodbye, Bowling Green, Ohio, and hello, Orlando, Florida.

The morning of the wedding, I joined the girls: the bride, her attendants, and Kelli, mother of the bride. Megan had reserved a suite at the Crowne Plaza in downtown Orlando and we were all having our hair done, as well as air-brushed make-up. What a special experience to share. It was there I learned Megan and Rico had received a message that morning saying the Caribbean cruise they were taking for their honeymoon would not be departing as scheduled.

We were all disappointed for Meg and Rico. However, the bride and groom were not overly upset by the news. Their spirit of joy was not to be stolen.

Watching her on the arm of my son, coming along the curving stone path that led into the patio room adjacent to the ballroom, and then out to the patio, brought tears of absolute pride and joy. Standing near the arch under a 100-year-old majestic, gnarled oak tree laden with moss, Rico and his dad, who was his best man stood watching. Soon tears were flowing from their eyes. So very touching. I actually think there were more men than women teary-eyed or crying.

The evening was filled with the three Ds: Dinner, Dancing, and Desserts. And laughter, lots of laughter. We all thought dinner couldn't be beat…then we spied the dessert tables laden with everything imaginable. I have never seen so many tantalizing and varied offerings, ever! Sandy and I were wondering just how many we could sample. Do we dare stuff our evening bags?

The high-energy chatter at the wedding was indicative of a joyous celebration of a new family just joined together. Everyone, young and old, was on the dance floor. The Pasambas are dancers for sure. Weddings are such a hope-filled time. If there is one thing these two families and friends have in common and do well, it is celebrating!

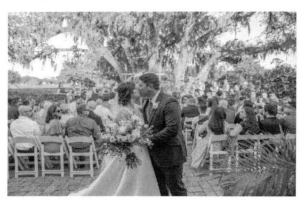

Sunday dawned and dramatic changes were on the horizon. Each of us began to receive texts about cancellations of our reservations for the week, along with worried texts from family and friends in California who were hearing concerning stories on the news. People hoarding food, toilet paper, and other paper products. San Francisco and Alameda counties were shutting down, only allowing grocery stores, banks, doctor's offices, and the post office to be open. The Bay area is known for its eccentricity, as well as its overreaction. Paranoia strikes deep. Meanwhile, in Florida, Walmart was running low on supplies, however, the local grocers like Publix were well stocked. It led us to believe the media was only focusing on the negative, and things weren't as bad as they seemed. We had no problem finding whatever we wanted.

Our vision of the days after the wedding had shrunk dramatically. As we began to consider alternatives to our original plans, we realized there were just not that many options.

Wedding guests from out of the country were urgently making changes to their flights to get home before the borders were closed and they would be trapped in Florida. The dream vacation location of many was suddenly undesirable.

Meanwhile, we were calmly planning our only day to see what we wanted to see. Glen, Barb, Sandy, and Jim wanted to go to Epcot. Rick and Kate wanted to go to Disney World, Hollywood, and Epcot. Sam, Christian, and I were joining grandkids from California and Kansas at Universal Studios. Christian had been to Disneyland and the Galaxy's Edge in California but had never been to Universal Studios.

We had a great time at Universal. There were seventeen of us anxious to enjoy ourselves. Three of my kids, their spouses, and my grandkids were all excited about the Harry Potter World venue. I suspect many people chose Disney World parks for their last day of enjoyment, but Universal still had plenty of visitors. There were no protocols in place, and masks were not the rule of the day at any of the facilities.

I lost my favorite hat which read, "Too Blessed to Be Stressed" on a ride I went on with Christian, but other than that, it was a successful "cousins" trip. You would never have known there was such a thing as the

Corona virus. Sunshine, food, rides, and laughter, that's what it was about.

Sandy, Jim, Glen, and Barb had gone to Epcot Center. Rick and Kate visited Disney World, Hollywood, and Epcot. They absolutely loved it. I think they would have spent the whole week there under normal circumstances.

The rest of the week was in limbo. It seems the only plan for the week that was not canceled was our alligator swamp boat ride on Monday. We piled onto the boat and away we went, searching for alligators.

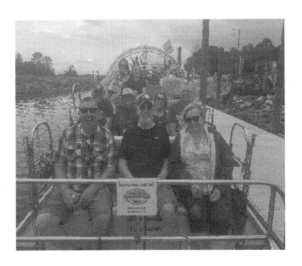

Many family members decided to change their flights and were gone by Tuesday rather than stay extra days as they had originally planned.

Christian's birthday was Tuesday. We were supposed to be at Disney World's Galaxy's Edge, followed by dinner at Disney Springs, with the famous Disney

Hat birthday cake. Disney announced on Monday they had decided to close Disney Springs immediately. So, again, we needed to be flexible and discover a new way to celebrate.

My brother Rick turned out to be the master chef on the trip. We invited the remaining family over for a swim and BBQ party: ribs, chicken, and all the side dishes we could find at the store. I was able to find a great cake and decorations last minute, and we celebrated his ninth birthday, Star Wars style.

Wednesday was a really tough day. Everyone was thinking they wanted to leave town. Fear of the possibility of closing the airport had Sandy concerned. We had tried Tuesday to reschedule with no luck. We tried again to reschedule our departure on Wednesday. After continuous attempts, we finally got through to Delta. There were not seven seats available. Everyone was leaving Florida like rats scurrying from a sinking ship. Finally, we threw in the towel and decided to stay until Saturday our original departure date.

Before everything closed, we had planned for my brothers and me to travel to Tampa to see the Yankees at spring training. Our son Chris and my granddaughter Taylor had driven down from Kansas to join us for her spring break, so instead, we decided on a trip to Daytona Beach. On the way, we stopped at Daytona Speedway, since one of our ideas had been to tour the track. That was for Jim. It was closed, so we stood outside the fenced-off area for photo ops.

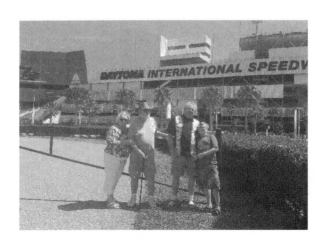

It was a Chamber of Commerce type day; sunshine, clear skies, and plenty of beach. Spring break was officially on, although the beaches were not overly crowded. Sunbathers, shoppers, and diners all enjoying what Florida is famous for. We went out to the end of the pier and had lunch at Joe's Crab Shack. It was the first time we had experienced a "virus" environment.

They had buckets placed on tables to signify non-occupancy and distancing. They would not seat our entire party of nine together or next to each other. My party of five was seated by a window, and as I gazed down, I saw dark shadows lurking in the waters below. I suddenly realized I was seeing sand sharks swimming very close to shore. People were in the shallow waters nearby, blissfully unaware of the danger as they frolicked in the waves.

Christian loved seeing the sharks and ran out onto the deck surrounding the restaurant. He was hoping we would go down for a closer look. Better judgment prevailed and we took photos instead. I look back on this moment often and think of how we were enjoying ourselves, naively unaware that we too were being stalked, by something every bit as deadly.

We spent the rest of our time wandering through the gift shops before heading back to our home base. Not exactly the vacation we had planned.

Chapter 4 - Hospital

I began feeling fatigued on Thursday afternoon while still in Florida. Really fatigued. I stumbled going up the stairs to our room, and lay there for a moment, short of breath. I had experienced this type of fatigue many times with Lupus, so I wasn't overly concerned. In addition, I probably wasn't over the lung infection I had contracted in January; a pretty common occurrence for me. We all went out to dinner and I began feeling a bit nauseous.

Friday morning dawned and I was the last one to rise. The last day of the "vacation" that wasn't. We had to do laundry, get rid of all the food in the fridge and pantry, clean the house, and pack. Our flight home was scheduled for 5:00 am the next morning and our driver was coming to pick up the girls, while the guys returned the rental van. We were all giddy with delight at getting out of Florida.

I came downstairs and sat at the breakfast table. Sipping on my coffee, I really began to feel nauseous.

I decided to go into the living room to be with Sam. As I sat across from him and was explaining to him how I felt, I lost consciousness.

I rolled off of the chair and onto the cold tile floor. "Sis, Sis, wake up." *Slap!* My loving brother hit me. I bet he enjoyed that. He tells me my color was green and he was very concerned. He had heard me crash onto the floor from the family room and came rushing in to see what had happened. As I regained consciousness, I asked, "Why am I lying on this cold floor?" Blood was pouring from my nose. It was broken and painful.

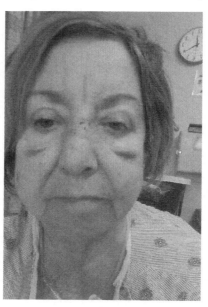

And all this before I'd had breakfast. As the day progressed, I decided to go visit Urgent Care. I knew they couldn't fix my broken nose, but I was definitely not feeling well.

The doctor was very gentle and confirmed my broken nose. I suspected I had pneumonia, as I am prone to have. His X-ray technician wasn't the best, or else I was a terrible patient. Either way, the X-rays didn't turn out, so he suggested I go to the hospital emergency room to get better ones. He also asked me if I had heard of hydroxychloroquine.

As I mentioned before, I have Lupus and had taken that drug for nearly twenty years, but was no longer using it. He then prescribed Z-Max, as well as the hydroxychloroquine, and off we went. By now it was early evening on Friday. There was no way I was going to sit for hours in an emergency room in Florida since I was leaving for California in a few hours. Besides, I would be in an emergency room surrounded by sick people, and I did not want to be exposed to Covid. I had my prescriptions, and thinking I had pneumonia, I was good to go.

Back to pack up and prepare for the early morning flight home. Thank goodness. The nightmare was finally going to be over. This long-anticipated vacation had turned into a journey of frustration and disappointment for all of us. No one was sorry to be leaving Orlando.

The airport was eerily empty. Delta had canceled 70% of their flights, which certainly helped explain why we could not get an earlier flight out. It felt like we were the last ones to leave Orlando. And no one was coming in. The flight was uneventful. Sandy and I did our sanitizing routine and offered others on the plane the opportunity to do the same but we had no takers.

There were few people wearing masks. Even the flight attendants were mask-less.

As soon as we arrived at my California home, where all my siblings had left their cars ten days earlier, hurried goodbyes and hugs were shared, and I went immediately to bed. I was still very fatigued. I'd been awake since 3:00 am Florida time. All I wanted was my own bed and a good night's sleep.

My daughter Missy, and my daughter-in-law Kelli, lovingly referred to as Nurse Kelli, had been urging me to go to the hospital emergency room. Both are medical professionals and they were really concerned. I promised to go the next day. I was just too tired to go today.

Sunday morning came and I was feeling better. I had spent the night in my own bed. It was still mid-morning and Sam asked if I wanted him to take me to the hospital. I called Sutter Roseville ER. When I told them my symptoms and that I had just returned from Florida, they told me NOT to come in; to call my doctor. Since it was Sunday, I knew he would not be in. I began to think I would wait and see my doctor on Monday. Missy insisted that CDC says to call the ER and tell them you are coming or call 9-1-1. She really wants me to go to the hospital emergency room. Obedience has never been my strong suit, so I disobeyed the instructions of the ER nurse's advice NOT to go to the ER.

About that time, my son Todd arrived. He was pretending to have just stopped by to see how I was. I knew his wife, "Nurse" Kelli, had sent him. I wasn't anticipating staying at the hospital, so I asked him if he would take me. That would allow Sam to be home with Christian. Todd was most accommodating. I didn't realize just how tired and weak I still was. Our chatter on the way to the hospital was not remarkable. Looking back, it could well have been our last conversation.

As we approached the Sutter Roseville Emergency Room entrance, I could see a drastic change. There had been construction going on before, but now, in addition to the metal fences cordoning off certain areas, there was just a small narrow path to the entrance to the ER. In the middle of the path, hospital personnel were pre-checking patients for entry. They asked a series of questions: Why are you here? What are your symptoms? We were not in that line long.

We were asked to return to the massive parking structure behind us. A portion had been "tented." It looked like how I imagined a military field medical setup would look.

They allowed Todd to wheel me to the entrance to the tents, but he was not allowed to enter. I'll never forget the look on his face at that time. This was unexpected for sure. We were both confused and a bit disappointed with the separation. Normally, when you go to the emergency room you sit and wait to be called for triage. Then, after a long wait, you are taken back to a room. Whoever brought you gets to accompany you for the long, three-hour-plus wait for tests, the diagnosis, and discharge. You were not alone to wait, wonder, and count the hours. I was truly expecting to go home that day.

The tent was partitioned off. The usual medical

personnel were there. One section was for taking your vitals and your history. The next partition was for evaluation.

The tent seemed to come alive upon my entry. Everyone seemed very interested in my history since I had just returned from Florida. Apparently, Florida was a hot spot for the Corona virus.

The usual long, drawn-out wait was dramatically short. I was whisked into an actual ER room. This was an isolation room especially for unconfirmed, but suspected, Covid patients.

My blood oxygen levels were low, so I was immediately placed "under a mask." Talk about painful. The attendant apparently had not read the part about my broken nose. Her ignorance of the fact was confirmed when she shoved what appeared to me to be a foot-long skewer with a cotton ball on the end up my nostril. My screaming, "My nose is broken," elicited an, "Oh, sorry."

This day was not unfolding as I had hoped and it was still early. Since I was in the actual hospital ER, I assumed my son could join me at this point. No, no, no. I was experiencing my first isolation. I'm hoping he's not worried. I am already planning on going home.

Because I was a "suspect," they were taking few chances. The equipment for chest X-rays and EKGs was brought into my room.

Lying there, no one to talk to, and people actually coming by my room peering in, I was beginning to feel like a specimen of sorts. The best part of having someone with you is not only someone to talk to, but also someone who can stand at the door, peer down the hall, catch the eye of a medical staffer, and ask when we might see the doctor, or tell them you need to go to the restroom.

Before the ER doctor came in, a nurse had come to check on me and mentioned that my lungs appeared to resemble photos of the lungs of Covid patients in Europe. That was soooo comforting. But I was impressed the hospital was that on top of things. All this Covid talk. At this point, I am still not concerned. I know, having self-diagnosed, that I have pneumonia and a broken nose. I didn't have any flu-like symptoms. Even if I did have Covid, it was only the flu. Or so I believed at the time. I would be going home soon.

Finally, the ER doctor arrived. He explained I had passed most of my tests. YES, I am thinking. I get to go home. However, he was still concerned over my losing consciousness and wanted to explore that issue more. He was admitting me to the hospital. He then introduced me to the doctor who would be my "hospitalist." All this new jargon. What ever happened to my own doctor taking care of me?

As the news spread, my family and friends still were not worried but relieved I was finally in the hospital. Some thought my breathing difficulties were because of my broken nose. At home, Sam, with tears in his eyes approached Christian and broke the news that I was staying at the hospital. Christian had never seen his Opa cry and began to think his Oma was not coming home. My poor sweet boys.

Of course, by the time I made it to my hospital

room, dinners had been ordered and were about to be delivered. That meant no Sunday Gravy for me. My alternative was a processed turkey sandwich on white bread. Not only unappetizing but also lacking in nutrition. Since I hadn't eaten since noon on Saturday, I was a bit disappointed. I just couldn't eat it.

Monday morning came early, as did the cold eggs. I was feeling nauseous and I had a fever. I have never taken a flu shot, due to my multiple immune system disorders and cannot remember the last time I had the flu either. They tell you to rest—all the while, every four hours, someone is checking your vitals. Add to that my teeny-tiny veins were not strong enough to withstand the antibiotics being pumped into me and "blew out" the IV three times. Having technicians digging around trying to find a useable vein was not my idea of a good time either. I kept telling them I did not possess one. They assured me when number two blew that they would do an ultrasound to find a stable one. They were wrong. They found the vein, but like all of my veins, it too was not strong and it blew. As I was not very clear-headed, I understand I conveyed I did not want IVs any longer. No one mentioned the use of IV delivery versus oral was much more effective. I needed the stronger doses of antibiotics to combat my pneumonia, so I resumed the torture.

When can I go home? I was sure I would be okay in my own bed where I could rest. All I need is rest. I was just so tired. And it was so boring. No visitors and I didn't watch TV that often unless it was a sporting event. March Madness, the college basketball classic had been canceled, much to my dismay. I could not fix my own meals and no one had given me a menu choice. Oh, what I would give for a Chick-fil-A sandwich.

I'm not sure what liquids were going into my veins but I was not feeling very alert. And did I mention fatigue? Very tired. I am wearing an oxygen mask and whenever I take it off to eat or go to the bathroom. my oxygen levels drop dramatically.

As I gazed out my window, I noticed a beautiful tree for me to enjoy. Thank you, God, for this reminder. I am feeling a bit depressed. I cannot go three minutes without oxygen. They have upped my oxygen to 5%.

They do blood draws between 3:00 am and 5:00 am so the doctors will have the results when they do their rounds. Some pleasant, smiley-faced person is always popping in. Where do they find such happy people? My all-time favorite test (not) is the blood gas test. They go directly into the artery to draw blood. Whenever I am watching a TV show where they mention the blood gas draw, I yell, "Don't let them do it."

I now have a cough and a fever. It's Tuesday. The hospitalist said on Sunday I would be here for a couple of days, so I am ready to go home now. Still waiting for the Covid test results. On Sunday they discussed getting setup and approved for local testing, but currently, everything has to go to San Diego. I continue to have a spiking fever. They do another wonderful nasal swab for Covid.

Wednesday is another day of disappointment. Besides getting another round of cold eggs for breakfast, I'm not getting better. I have resigned myself to the fact that I am not here for a Michelin dining experience and the priority is getting me well. Being isolated from family and friends since Sunday is hard, and talking makes my oxygen levels go down. Yesterday, the doctor told Nurse Kelli he was considering letting me go home today. That's not going to happen. This pneumonia is seriously kicking my butt.

It was difficult for me to talk. I had oxygen running 24/7 and talking made me tired, as well as short of breath.

I tried to avoid the news as much as possible. There was such a small chance of getting Covid, and it was only a bad flu anyway, right? The news is primarily focused on the negative side. Cynical would best describe my view of the news. Believe half of what you see and none of what you hear. Stories would later be determined to be half-truths filled with relentless negative suppositions. Fear of the pandemic was growing. Conflicting reports surfaced daily. I had lost confidence that any news station was credible; not CNN, not Fox, and definitely not the BBC. The media had long ago abandoned real reporting. Sensational and misleading headlines replaced factual, believable reports.

What if I died? My grandson Christian would lose yet another important figure in his short life. He just turned nine, and he has had so many challenges to face already. After all, he didn't choose his parents and he didn't choose to live with his grandparents. I thought about how old I was and that I would probably not witness his young adult years. It was unlikely I would meet his future spouse or children. His children would have no grandparents to take them to Disneyland when they turned ten; a tradition we had started with our first grandchild. Upon turning double-digits they got a trip, without their parents, to Disneyland, as well as California Adventure for five days. They chose all the restaurants and meals except for our traditional Rain Forest dinner. So sad it has closed now. Odd the things you think about when facing such uncertainty!

Is it unnatural to not fear death? I do not want to die, but I am not afraid of it. God is not a deal maker, and since I have nothing to bargain with, what are my options? And so, I wait.

I was being treated with hydroxychloroquine, zinc, azithromycin, as well as supplemental oxygen. After four days, my oxygen supplement needs to be escalated considerably. As I was one of the "pioneer" Covid patients, there were no established protocols, and doctors and nurses alike were pressed into utilizing practices and medications not guaranteed to be effective in combatting this disease.

It is March 26, 2020. My sister had sent an email the night before. "Hey sis, didn't know if you were taking calls. Hope you know something soon." An emoji with a smile and three small hearts were included. Me: "No not taking calls. Hoping to hear today. I will let you know."

What is happening now? The nurse is telling me I am being moved to the Covid Intensive Care floor. I now have a Rapid Response Team taking care of me. Somehow, I feel relieved that I am getting such focused care. That can't be bad. But this is all happening too fast. I was not expecting this. I should be going home.

They lost my breakfast. I am sure it was cold anyway. The doctor just confirmed I have Covid. Looking back, I cannot believe how calm I was.

My oxygen supplement requirements began to climb. The oxygen mask is no longer effective. They want to place me on a ventilator and they are asking me to sign papers regarding end-of-life measures. There is no one here I can discuss this with. In retrospect that was a good thing. They say ignorance is bliss. In this case, it was absolutely true. I had no idea that going on the ventilator was best known as life support. This machine was going to perform all my life-sustaining functions for me. Still, I had no thoughts of dying. Not one. Not watching the news sometimes pays off. I had avoided the crippling fear so many were beginning to feel.

It was unknown to me at this point that it was likely I would not survive. My last post to friends on Facebook was, "The battle is on."

I had no idea how true that statement would be. There is a lot to be said for a positive attitude. For the next two weeks, I was heavily sedated, unaware of what was happening with my friends and family, while doctors and nurses worked around the clock to save my life. A repeat chest X-ray revealed substantial worsening of bilateral air spaces typical of severe Covid disease. The steroid methyl-prednisone was added to the arsenal of medications.

The medical staff contacted Sam daily. The reports were overwhelming him. Not understanding the terminology, he soon turned to Kelli and had her interact with the medical personnel and decipher all the updates. Meanwhile, he buried himself in homeschooling Christian and arranging for Zoom music lessons and Karate.

My poor sweet Sam. He prayed constantly. He knew the possibilities, as well as the probabilities, that our holding hands, snuggling, or kissing may never happen again. He refused to accept them as reality. He does not hang out with the guys anymore. His sole purpose in life seems to be making me happy and being with me every day. There is not a selfish bone in his body. He has always put others before himself, especially me. Most of his thoughts are centered on what he can do to make others happy or their lives better. How did I get so fortunate? And now he was alone waiting to see how this crazy Corona-Covid virus was going to affect our lives.

One week after I was admitted to the hospital, my brother Rick and my sister Sandy were diagnosed with Covid. Rick was placed immediately on a ventilator. He was in a small hospital near his home near Nevada City. My brother Glen was to enter the hospital days later. He required oxygen therapy and was not placed on a ventilator, although his oxygen levels and lack of being aware of his surroundings left a lot to be worried about. Covid brain is real.

Imagine, all four of us in the hospital at the same time, battling an unknown virus that the medical profession was just beginning to grapple with. Our families were in disbelief. Each family had a unique battle of its own. A medical war raging on four fronts.

It was early on and hysteria was running rampant. The entire medical profession was in uncharted waters, not sure what worked, and finding there are so many variables. A virus like this had never been seen before. I was fortunate to have had a wonderful team of medical specialists who worked tirelessly and with passion. I had pneumonia, as well as Covid. Coupled with my underlying immune system disorders; my prospects of survival were not high.

News of my illness spread rapidly. I was on multiple prayer chains. A personal friend, Claire, and a business colleague, Kelly, kept everyone updated on Facebook. Approximately 10,000 people were praying for me worldwide. Claire posted a different photo and an update every day, making it personal for those who I had not met but were praying for me.

My neighbors were so supportive of Sam and Christian; grocery shopping, games, and books for Christian. Always available to help out. Few people expected me to survive, including my boy, Christian. He says he would look out the window for several hours each day to check and see if I was coming home. He could not go to Karate, piano lessons, baseball practice, or see any of his friends because of Covid. His life had come to a screeching halt and his aunt, uncles, and Oma were all in the hospital.

While in ICU on the ventilator, I was "flipped." That's a process known as proning, where my bed is actually turned over so that I am on my stomach. It boosts oxygen levels temporarily. With the masks, tubes, wires, and the equipment I was hooked up to, I cannot imagine what it looked like or how it was even possible.

Ever so slowly, I become vaguely aware of the light. I hear voices, though they sound faint and far away. I hear they are going to try to take me off of the ventilator. Try? Is this something that may not work? How do they take you off of a ventilator? Is it in my chest? Is it a surgical procedure? Where are the people I can ask? I'm lying here alone with so many questions. Then I notice the ceiling tiles. They are moving. Could that be it? When the tiles are centered over me the machine will be lifted?

Time is dragging by. No one is coming in to see me. What's this? My tongue has found this "thing" in my throat. There is very little space between it and my throat. As my tongue feels around, I began to get frightened. I notice I can get my tongue behind this thing and press a bit. If I keep my tongue there, I will be able to continue breathing, but if I'm not able to do this, I will choke to death. Please, please, won't someone come into my room? I dare not close my eyes or go to sleep. Help me.

It is then I notice my arms are restrained. I could pull out my tubes, so I have been bound up for my own safety. I cannot use a call button. I can't talk. I can't call for help. I am actually terrified. Isolated, alone. No way to communicate or ask for help. I couldn't speak. Somebody, PLEASE come in my room.

The next thing I am aware of is being in a dark room and a nurse giving me ice chips. My throat is very sore, and the chips are so soothing. I need more. Can I have more? For the first twenty-four hours after removing the ventilator, they limit the amount of chips I can have. It is a precaution to keep me from choking. They cannot allow me to self-administer the chips because if I began to choke, they wouldn't reach me in time. In order to come into my room, they must first don disposable gowns, booties, masks, and gloves. Again, I can't sleep as I await my next dose of ice. My throat is on fire and the soothing flow of relief from the ice does not last long.

When I am finally able to "speak," I find I cannot. My voice is gone. I still have no way to communicate. I hand signal for something to write on. They find a small board and pen for me. Oh, no. My hands are so shaky and I am so weak, I can't write. Focus, Lynda, focus. I slowly get the pen to touch the pad. My shaking continues. After a few frustrating attempts, I finally get it down. "Can I go home?"

"When can I go home?" and "I want to go home" became my daily request. I was convinced if I stayed in the hospital, I would die, but if I was allowed to go home, I would be ok. It may seem like an unreasonable fear, but not to me. People die in hospitals. I could get another illness.

They moved me to another room in ICU; my fifth room change. This room was equipped with "jet propulsion" blowers. In other words, extremely loud blowers were oxygenating my environment. My hearing has not totally returned to normal as a result of the loud noise.

A wonderful nursing assistant asks me what I would like as my first food or drink. Hmm. Remember, I haven't eaten in about three weeks. Endless possibilities. A medium-rare steak? A Chick-fil-A sandwich? Mexican or Chinese food? Boy, that ice cream was wonderful. Yes, I chose ice cream. Popsicles also became a favorite as my throat constantly cried out to be soothed.

When I was taken off of the ventilator, my family had decided that perhaps I should not be told about my other siblings. Thank goodness Glen didn't get the message and kept me informed about Rick and Sandy with his daily calls. Unfortunately, with my weak voice and shortness of breath, I was not able to be a good communicator, but I listened as he updated me on the conditions of my other two siblings, as well as how he was doing. I was unaware that every one of them had entered the hospital after I did until I spoke to him.

Sandy and Rick could not communicate. Both were in ICU on ventilators. At one point, Glen reported that both had taken a turn for the worse. I am praying often for my family. I feel so helpless. Both Glen and Sandy are here in the same hospital. So close, but yet so far. Never once did I even consider that we would not all be together soon, sharing our experiences, and resuming Sibling Sundays.

I have a tablet in my room. I am just too tired to use it. My body is weak. People are going by my window, waving and giving me a thumbs up! I am a survivor. It has been so long since I have had human contact. I just want a hug and to hold someone's hand.

It's extremely lonely. In recent years, a wave of studies has documented some incredible emotional and physical health benefits that come from touch. This research is suggesting that touch is truly fundamental to human communication, bonding, and health.

(www.greatergood.berkeley.edu, *Hands on Research: The Science of Touch,* Dacher Keltner, September 29, 2010.)

I was surrounded by an entire hospital of people who had a variety of protection on. Some had a mask on, as well as a transparent shield. Some wore "beekeepers" head gear. All wore gloves, booties, and were covered from head to toe in disposable gear. Very few touched me. I even had to pull myself up in bed. All this gear was removed and not worn outside my room. It was a bit disconcerting knowing the people who were in charge of my survival knew so little about the virus and its transmission.

I cannot sleep and wind up constantly channel surfing. I find such interesting offerings: *My 600 lb. Life*, *Housewives of Miami*, *New Jersey*, and every major city in America, and the endless news. The same reports on every channel. Why so many news channels if they all repeat the same words and stories?

Have you ever experienced hallucinations? It is a perception of having seen, heard, touched, tasted, or smelled something that was not there. Hallucinations are one of the many "gifts" of Covid. Remember when I was desperate for ice? My Covid brain had the nurse show me how to make the ice pitcher come to me, once my twenty-four hours were up. Which meant I did not have to wait for medical personnel to come in. They kept that at a minimum anyway. It gets better. I had these amazing straws and utensils to eat with. When I focused my eyes on, say a drink container, I could move it closer to me. Since I was too weak to place the straws in my drinks, the nursing assistants had already placed them in the container for me before exiting my room.

The plates and silverware were specialized, as well as disposable. They also magically moved upon concentration. What great technology! However, there was no heat retention in my food and drink, and reheating in the microwave was forbidden. Even my morning coffee was cold. It was not until about six months after my discharge that I discovered this was not reality. Except for the cold food. During a time of deep reflection, I could no longer visualize this extraordinary technology and slowly realized, after confirming with hospital personnel, that it had never existed. A pretty disturbing turn of events.

Discussion of my discharge had included the suggestion I consider going to a rehabilitation hospital. The mere thought of being placed in a convalescent hospital with potential Covid patients was not appealing to me. I had seen enough television reports regarding those places in New York and New Jersey. Nope, not going there. No one knew if I would be immune or if it was possible to get Covid again.

The caveat was that I had to remain isolated and in quarantine for fourteen days after discharge if I went directly home. I would get to sleep in my own bed at long last. My sweet husband could not join me, hug me, or touch me. However, just the thought of seeing him and Christian every day and being in my own home where I felt safe and secure was so uplifting. They were also assigning a home health nurse, as well as a physical therapist to visit me during this time. It was an easy decision for me.

Chapter Five – Going Home

It was a gorgeous, sunny California day. There was hardly a cloud in the sky. It seemed like it was designed just for me. My son Todd was there to take me home. I am told he left for the hospital almost immediately upon hearing I would be discharged. He waited patiently for hours. He was not allowed inside the hospital and communication for discharge on a Saturday was less than efficient. It was to be my first breath of fresh air in weeks.

In my last few days in the hospital, I thought of breathing in the air and being free from the tubes, the prods and pokes, and the daily shots in the stomach, as well as the every-four-hour visits. I would put it all behind me. It was a beautiful Saturday and the streets were practically deserted. As I searched the skies, taking in the sun and clouds floating overhead, I could feel something was missing. It is the day before Easter. No traffic. The streets are deserted. No cars in the parking lots of the shopping centers. Where are the shoppers?

Not even any bikers are out. Much had transpired while I was in my drug-induced twilight. Businesses were closed. Masks were required. Fear and uncertainty were beginning to creep into the fabric of society. It was like entering the Twilight Zone. It had an eerie feeling to it. But I was so happy to be going home. I would be safe there. Todd reminded me that a lot had changed in the weeks since I came back from Florida

I had my walker, my oxygen tanks, and my gratitude to take home with me. My Bernese Mountain dog had missed me along with Sam and Christian. My dog Bernie was so excited he almost got tangled up in my cannula. That's the little plastic "hose" with a connection placed in your nose to deliver the oxygen.

It was not a normal homecoming. I could not hug Todd, Sam, or Christian. I got to switch oxygen tanks from the portable I came home from the hospital with, to the one large tank that had been delivered earlier in the day. It came with a very, very long "hose." I went immediately to my "isolation" room. I had to wear a mask…in my own home.

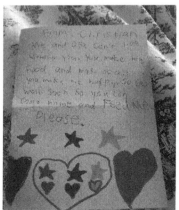

Christian made a get-well card for me.

"from Christian. Me and Opa can't live without you. You make me food and most of all you make me happy. So, get well soon. Come home and feed me. Please."

Underneath were stars and a big heart. Made my homecoming sweet!

Sam made sure everything was sterile. He had fresh sheets on the bed and a bed tray on which to serve my food. He even sanitized the mail. Reality began to set in. I would be here for fourteen days. Living with people in the same house, but unable to hold, touch, hug or kiss. No contact. I began the countdown that very day. I missed Sam's touch so much.

All of Sam's actions reminded me of why I fell in love and married him in the first place. It seems so long ago.

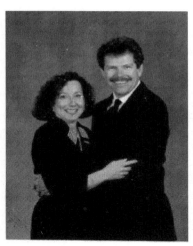

After having been divorced for nearly twelve years and dating all the wrong men, I was resigned to not dating. Period. My boys were three and five when their dad left. Now they were teenagers. Their childhood was basically fatherless, so I had little motivation to complicate my life with a husband.

Like my siblings, I had married my high school sweetheart several years after graduation. Ironically, Sam had done the same. Neither marriage worked out well other than producing a total of three boys and three girls between us.

One Sunday, after having spent a week in Washington D.C. on business, I drug my jet-lagged body to church. I had a choice between attending services and going to bible study. As tired as I was, I thought perhaps I would fall asleep during the service. At least in bible study people would be talking and keep me awake.

It was there I met Sam. Like me, he had been divorced a long time. He had had a dream where one of his closest friends told him he needed to go to church THAT Sunday. Why he picked the church I was attending, and how we came to meet, is a mystery. This was a large church, but meet we did.

I felt he added insight and lively conversation during the study, but when it was over, I headed straight for my car. Sam was behind me, walking in the same direction. He began asking questions about the class and the church as this was his first time attending, and so I stopped to chat. The small talk became a bit more personal as he asked about my profession and introduced me to his two daughters, who had just walked up to him. I gave him the forensic once over. He was attractive and appeared to be a bit younger than me. That is always a plus as women are supposed to edge out men in longevity. He had a good job, but what really intrigued me was his confident, relaxed manner, his spirit, and the fact he had raised four children by himself for the past eight years. I was smitten.

Almost as soon as I arrived home, I phoned a good friend and declared I had met the man I was going to marry. I had never felt such a strong, immediate attraction before. Imagine how I was feeling when he did not call me until Thursday night of that week. After a two-hour conversation, he still had not asked me out. What is with this guy? It took him two weeks to ask me to go on a motorcycle ride with him.

We had stopped to look at the lake. It was early evening and the sky was filled with soft pastel blues and multiple shades of salmon. We had taken our helmets off and were talking when he suddenly turned his head to comment. His lips brushed mine lightly. Wow! I can hardly wait until we actually kiss! That pretty much sealed the deal though. Learning more about him, I knew he was sincere, honorable, and kind. It didn't hurt that he had really nice "biker buns" from riding motorcycles. I knew Sam was the kind of man who would be there for me no matter what. Trustworthy.

When you know it; you know it. We were engaged and subsequently married six months later. He suggested we wait a year, however, when I explained to him if we waited a year, I was sure I would have found a reason NOT to marry him, he happily said I DO.

After the evening, candlelight ceremony, I tossed white, lacy leggings to two bridesmaids and announced we were riding to the reception on the backs of motorcycles. We hiked up our dresses and away we went. In case you were wondering these were not Harley Fat

Boys, but big touring motorcycles, built for a comfortable ride and long-distance travel.

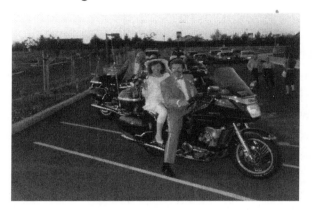

On our first-month anniversary, I received a gold foil box at my downtown office. It contained a dozen long-stemmed chocolate chip cookies. Such a "sweet surprise." His philosophy was that waiting a year to celebrate an anniversary was much too long, so we celebrated monthly. All the while opening doors for me, holding my hand wherever we went, and sharing a light kiss after saying Grace at our evening meal. Such a lucky girl.

In usual Sam-like fashion, he adapted to our altered circumstances. Just happy that I was home where he could take care of me. Christian, however. seemed wary of me, as if he didn't know just what was happening. I learned later that he, along with many of our family and friends, had prayed for, but not totally expected, this day to happen. Each morning after I came home, he would wake up and peek into my room to see if I was still breathing. It was such a terrible time for everyone, but especially for a nine-year-old.

Christian first came to stay with us when he was two. Child Protective Services called us and asked if we had a grandson named Christian, and were we willing to come to pick him up. If not, they were preparing to put him in Foster Care. I had seen him twice in his lifetime. Once at the hospital when he was born, and again about a year later. The environment he was living in was so distressing, I could not go back. Sam and I took about five seconds to respond to the caller.

Where do we pick him up? We arrived to find a determined little boy with a bag packed waiting for two people he did not know. I recall how stoic he was as we drove away. No tears. No apparent fear. Almost everything he had with him had to be sanitized or thrown out.

No one from CPS was at the address we were given, only his mother and one of the people she lived with. Fourteen people in a three-bedroom house. We had no idea what we were to do. What if he needed medical care? Where is the authorization for us to care for him? What if we had not shown up or someone else took him? Days went by before we finally got a return phone call from a caseworker.

I could go into what a horribly dysfunctional system CPS is, but that would take an entire book on its own. Suffice it to say, the only joy was in discovering what a gift we had been given.

Christian's mom entered a treatment facility, and after a few months, she came to live with us. We had hoped she would be able to get a job and make a home for herself and Christian.

Eventually, Sam and I decided we would retire and make our lifelong plan of traveling for a few years a reality. Christian's mom had lived with us for almost one and a half years, but had made no progress in securing a stable future. We gave her six months' notice to make arrangements to move out on her own. Of course, we had concerns that she would be able to create a safe and loving environment for him, but we had hoped this would spur her into action and motivate her. She had the tools but would she have the desire?

We loved traveling. We had picked up two of our grandsons in Kansas and traveled to Mt. Rushmore. From there we went to the Black Hills, Yellowstone, the Grand Tetons, and a famous skate park in Denver. After returning them to Kansas, we went on to visit friends in Michigan and our granddaughter at college in Ohio.

It was while there we received an invitation to return to California for a family trip to Disneyland. I had developed what appeared to be an undiagnosable medical condition, so we thought returning to my doctors was a good idea. While back in California, Christian came for a visit and has remained with us since that time. He had been with us nearly five years when Covid struck.

What a gift he is! Not only kind. He is funny, intelligent, creative, compassionate, and always wakes up happy. Unlike many "only children," he does not need entertainment. His imagination is limitless and he is a joy to be around.

Isolation at home was not that easy. I had to remain

in my room and bathroom area only. Sam would mask up and bring in a tray and leave it. I had a chair and a bed. I needed the walker to get to the bathroom. Sam and Christian had to remain socially distanced and masked. No hugs allowed.

On Monday after I was discharged, I saw my home health nurse. She checked my lungs, vital signs, and generally assessed how I was doing. She let me know when my physical therapist was supposed to come. The therapist never arrived. I spoke by phone to my home health nurse about it later that week and she said she would follow up and see to it that she came the following Monday. I was in such a hurry to recover. Why wasn't everyone else on board? It seems the PT assigned to me was so fearful of Covid, that she sat outside my home in her car and had the nurse "test me." I suggested she leave my exercise information on the porch and not come back. I had little patience for someone who was willing to be paid for not doing her job.

Sam was busy keeping Christian occupied and preparing meals. Christian was sad that I was uncomfortable. He is such an incredible young man. He tells me it was hard and he tried to pretend everything was okay. Wearing a mask in the house made him uncomfortable too. My voice was so weak, Sam could not always hear me if I needed something. He and Christian came up with a clever solution. Christian had a toy police bullhorn that made siren noises. I tied it to my walker and whenever I needed anything, I just pushed the button. It was so fun!

Meanwhile, my thoughts were on my siblings. I

began every morning with a prayer for each one of them. Again, I wondered how did this happen? Why all four of us? Was it my fault? Am I the reason they are in the hospital? Did I carry the virus and pass it to them? Why didn't our spouses get sick? So many questions with no answers.

Chapter Six – Sibling Stories

The day I went to ICU with the confirmation of Coronavirus, Rick had begun running a fever. He was awaiting a return call from his doctor and watching *Gunsmoke* reruns. Three days later he was admitted to the hospital.

While I was in a regional trauma center, he was hospitalized in a small hospital near his home in Nevada City, California. He had begun his week feeling tired but shrugged it off. Later in the week he wasn't feeling well and decided to have a Covid test. The results would take ten days. Really! How much sicker could you get waiting? On Sunday night, March 31, 2020, he went to the hospital. At first, they were going to send him home, but then decided he should stay.

Shortly after admission, he was placed on a ventilator in ICU. This was an unusual step, but so little was known about the virus that there were no prescribed protocols established about how to combat serious cases of the virus, so a ventilator was frequently employed. The prognosis was not good. DNR papers were being required. Kate had been told he was probably not going to make it.

Kate was terrified. She and Rick had only been married seven years. He is undoubtedly the love of her life. They created a custom home in a panoramic mountain setting. Future retirement plans were exciting dreams with travel at the top of the list. Rick had retired from the probation department and was patiently waiting for Kate to join him. Fear gripped her heart. Now, what would happen? How would she go on? You begin to wonder, worry, and imagine what the future may hold. It is a dark place. She was home, in quarantine, isolated and alone.

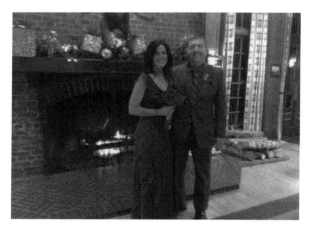

Sandy and Rick entered the hospital on the same date. Sandy went into a local hospital in Auburn, California, but was subsequently transferred to the ICU unit at the hospital I was in. They were soon responding to treatment well and the prognosis was improving.

Then, without warning, they both took a turn for the worse, each experiencing a cytokine storm. It's a complication in Covid that triggers your immune system to flood your bloodstream with inflammatory proteins called cytokines. It can destroy tissues and damage your organs. This was not good news. What a true roller coaster of emotions.

They both began to show evidence of kidney failure. The doctors were considering dialysis for Rick when, once again, his kidneys began to function properly. During his time on the ventilator, the doctors had to paralyze his diaphragm to allow the ventilator to breathe for him. He had been the healthiest and strongest sibling but now was having to fight for his life.

He was somewhat of a celebrity patient at this small local hospital. There was no Covid unit. His doctor conferred with the doctors at my hospital regarding treatments. Eventually, Rick came off the ventilator. Everyone was so grateful that the worst had passed. But, of course, his recovery was not easy.

He was in quite a fog. He seemed very confused and disoriented. He had a feeding tube in place as he could not swallow. In his confusion, he tried to pull it out. When the hospital staff went to reinsert the tube, they punctured his lung. They had to intubate him four times. Eventually, they placed a "peg tube" in his stomach as a replacement for the feeding tube.

His doctor was a huge support. He allowed Kate and Katie, his daughter, to visit. First, it was via phone with them being outside the window but gradually progressed to actual in-person visits.

Like me, Rick had hallucinations. His family was concerned he might not recover from the neurological issues they were seeing. One thing for sure, until he was home, they could not be confident he would be okay.

Being in isolation at home gave me plenty of time to think. I began reflecting on our childhood years. Rick was the baby. With five and a half years between us, and our older siblings out of the house with families of their own, we were left to grow up together. I became the resident big sister.

I always felt I needed to protect him, and yet, he was bigger than I was. He was the tallest one in the family besides my dad. Despite the age difference, we got along great. We both loved being outdoors, riding bikes, then later on riding mopeds.

I sometimes thought I should have been a boy. I will never forget how unhappy my mom was every Christmas. I would ask Santa for adventuresome sporting items. Instead, I would get a doll—every year. I did not play with dolls, so that was a problem. Occasionally Dad would take us fishing or to the hot rod races on Friday nights. On the first day of summer vacation after his kindergarten year, Rick challenged me to a bike race down our neighbor's very steep driveway. He was in the lead but I was gaining on him. He looked back to see how close I was and *BAM*, over he went. I was trying hard not to run over him, but I applied the brakes just as my wheels were riding over his body. Broken collar bone. And just like that, summer play was over.

Living in the country there was always an abundance of stray dogs and cats for us to enjoy. Summers were hot, so one day we decided to give the latest batch of kittens a bath in a huge metal tub filled with water. There were too many kittens to carry at once, so we each decided to take them one at a time to the tub. It didn't take long for us to realize kittens do not swim. I think Rick was traumatized for life. He, like my brother Glen, is a sensitive guy.

After high school, Rick joined the Air Force, went to college, graduated with a degree in Criminal Justice, and began his career in law enforcement. He, like Glen and Sandy, moved with his wife to the historic and picturesque foothills of the Nevada City area to raise their girls, Katie and Alison.

Sandy, on the other hand, had been checked out and sent home from the local hospital emergency room in Auburn, Ca. So little was known. It almost seemed like medical personnel were reluctant to admit someone without proof of Covid. She was eventually readmitted to that same hospital. Not long after, she was transferred to the hospital I was in. Her family was encouraged since I had been on the ventilator for two weeks by this time and was holding my own. However, the statistics and national news regarding survival rates for patients on ventilators were very worrisome.

Her husband Jim had been the one everyone was concerned about. He had a serious lung disease. Would he be next? He thought Sandy would be okay if they would just send her home and let him take care of her. Was it denial or just a lifelong partner wanting her by his side to love and care for her?

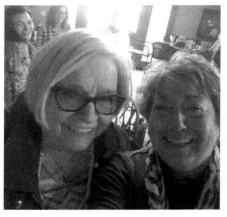

Sandy and I had grown so close over the past few years. I love thinking about it since it was not always the case. Being compared to my sister all my life was a reminder of how different the two of us were. I was constantly asked by my mother, "Why can't you be like your sister?" My thought always was, because I am not, I am me.

Sandy took after the German side of the family, big bones and solid, while I quit growing around the age of twelve. I topped out at four foot eleven and skinny. I'm still the same height but have managed to gain some weight. One of my aunt's used to laugh when she recalled that at age five, I resembled an orangutang. Ouch! I definitely do not have that issue today.

Sandy was full of life and everyone enjoyed being around she and Jim. I, on the other hand, always felt like a square peg in a round hole.

If there was one thing my sister dearly loved, it was her grandchildren. She had lunch with her granddaughter regularly and, much to her amusement and sometimes shock, Skyler shared every detail of her life. You could tell how proud she was that her granddaughter was so open in sharing.

She married her high school sweetheart. Jim was

the football-playing drag racer, and Sandy was the blonde song leader. Jim's love for cars and enjoyment of driving led to a successful career with UPS. Together, they were a light-hearted, fun-loving couple who enjoyed many friendships throughout their lives.

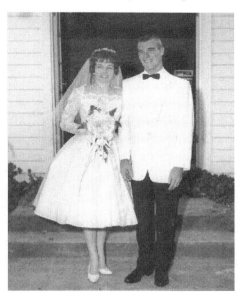

Growing up in Northern California in Sacramento County's rural area of Orangevale, made Christian Valley near Auburn, California attractive to Sandy and Jim. It was there they raised their children, Wendy and Jim Jr.

Sandy was not the athletic type. Oh no. Weight Watchers was a part of her life in an on-again, off-again sort of way. She would achieve success, then food won out, then back to Weight Watchers. It's no wonder she found managing her weight a challenge. She had so many friends and social lunches on a regular basis.

Who had time to count points? We both joined the new Weight Watchers in June of 2020 in anticipation of the wedding, and hoping not to have to resort to "tent dressing."

Sandy was a bit conservative. Although never one to miss out on an opportunity for fun, she had her limits. She could be the life of the party, but she was not about to embarrass herself and throw caution to the wind. She found a way to put levity in almost any situation and it was natural, sometimes self-deprecating, humor. Often described as an amazing woman, she was rarely negative. She was also much more private.

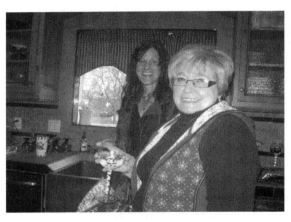

The last sibling to enter the hospital was Glen, my older brother. He and my sister-in-law had decided they should go in for testing. The hospital kept my brother and sent Barbara home alone.

All of us had one common symptom. Shortness of breath. Glen was placed on supplemental oxygen but did not have to be placed on the ventilator. I am grateful for that. Barbara was surprisingly calm and confident her beloved husband of fifty-nine years would be all right.

Glen found time to face time or call me daily while he was in the hospital and I was off the ventilator. He was frustrated that his oxygen levels were taking their time settling down. Good one day, not so good the next, but eventually he stabilized and was able to go home.

Glen, whose nickname is Corky, is the oldest. Sandy often commented on his silken, silver-shaded hair. Isn't it funny that siblings always seem to find they got left out in the gene pool in one way or another?

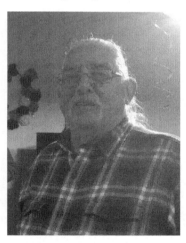

Being sentimental, he vowed not to cut his hair until his grandson returned from his four-year enlistment with the Air Force. Apparently, Glen never considered his grandson would choose the Air Force as a career and re-enlist.

Currently, he is still chopping wood for the fire,

living on his mini-farm in Newcastle, and socializing with family and friends. I can hardly believe he is eighty years old. If there is anybody with a heart bigger than my brother Glen, I have never met them.

Have you ever met someone and immediately felt like he was a friend? That's my brother. If you've been introduced to him, you are a new friend. He remembers your name and everything you've ever shared with him. If you mention you need something or are looking to buy something, he immediately takes it on as a project. And even though he is known to be cranky at times, he generally has a big smile and an easy laugh waiting.

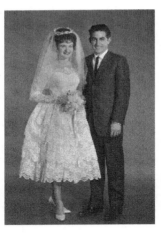

Like Sandy, he also married his high school sweetheart, Barbara, and immediately began his family; first Michael and then LeAnn.

Glen worked in the aerospace industry. He was so well-liked and respected there that after he retired and was given a great retirement party, he was called back three times, and given three more retirement parties. We all think he went back to work just so they would throw more parties.

He kept busy with Barbara's florist shop. For years there were trips to the flower mart in San Francisco. The shop was filled with a variety of unique gifts and plants and her creative skills as a florist were in demand. He regularly volunteered to serve those in need in his community and sang in a barbershop quartet, as well as at church.

Growing up, I felt so close to him, though we were eight years apart in age. Even then, he had a constant smile and an enthusiasm for life. I felt important to him. He would take me on rides to the store. Being small anyway, I would sit on my legs to make myself look taller, and hope that people thought I was his girlfriend.

My high school years were difficult. The teenage years, hormones, and, as my mother used to call my BULLHEADEDNESS, led to many differences of opinion, but I knew I could talk to my brother and Barbara about my relationship troubles with my mom. As I look back, I was one of those kids who was lucky my mother let me live. No matter what, Glen was there for me.

Rock and Roll was truly "rockin" back then. We had a "hi-fi" and plenty of vinyl records, and we would dance, dance, dance. It is my favorite childhood memory. We still dance today.

I missed him so much when he got married. It was the beginning of my loneliest time as a child.

Chapter 7 - Recovery

Settling into isolation, I had a wonderful view from my bedroom window and looked forward to mornings when I could prop up in bed and look out at the peaceful view. It was also a time of reflection. Comforting childhood memories, as well as more recent Sibling Sunday dinners, came to mind.

We had the perfect backdrop for those Sundays; the home we all grew up in. The home where family Christmases, Easter Sunday picnics, and Sunday dinners all began.

My husband and I decided to help my parents transition into their dream retirement facility. They had purchased their home in 1949 and we had all grown up there. Even though we had a comfortable home with a pool, spa, rock firepit, diving rock, and waterfall, we decided we would purchase their home so they could make their move.

It needed a lot of work, so we chose to rent our home out and live in theirs. The plan was they could have their house back if the new living arrangements were not what they had hoped, and we would return to our comfy house in the burbs.

Obviously, they enjoyed their new home and new friends. We got comfortable living on 1.3 acres in the country that was only a twenty-minute drive to either Galleria in our area, easy freeway access, one mile to the American River where bike trails and kayaking awaited us, and three miles to Folsom Lake for boating.

The day after I got home was Easter. Our neighbors had left an Easter basket for Christian on the front porch. That porch became central to my recovery. No one could come into the house, so they left packages almost daily.

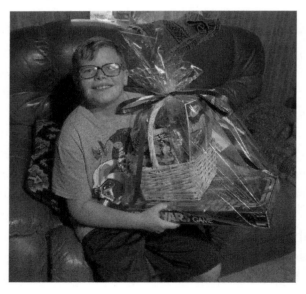

My son Todd brought over a traditional Easter dinner. What a wonderful day it was. My thoughts often turned to rejoining the human race once again. At the end of fourteen days, I could not only hug Sam and Christian, but I could also join them for meals, go outside and breathe the air I was allergic to. It was spring and everything was blooming. I couldn't wait. I was grateful I no longer had to have daily shots in my stomach to reduce the possibility of blood clots, or finger pricks to check for diabetes.

I spent my days resting, reading, and coloring in my adult coloring book. That, and consuming popsicles...lots of popsicles. My throat was very sore from the tubing in the hospital.

My voice was very weak, as was my physical strength. It doesn't take long for muscles to atrophy. Not to mention, I wasn't exactly a healthy specimen before Covid. Getting tied up with my walker and my oxygen hose was a frequent occurrence. Such were my early days in quarantine. Grateful to be home. So grateful. There is something very calming about being in familiar surroundings. That, and the knowledge I was not going to die. The entire time I was in the hospital I was not sure I would be coming home, thus my constant request to be released. I was positive that once I came home, I would not die.

I had survived the virus, while many others, especially on the East Coast, had not. I had been the first sibling to enter the hospital and now I was home. Each day I imagined how it would be on Day 14. I envisioned taking my initial walk outside. I would go to the first speed bump on our road and then turn around. It seemed like a conservative distance for my first outing.

When channel surfing, I found the news in the world was particularly ugly. It seems being an election year had tainted every action. A never-ending onslaught of negative, fear-filled, rhetoric. I recall seeing an East Coast story about a Covid ward. Television cameramen and reporters were interviewing medical staff and showing bed after bed of patients, side by side in a room. There was a hospital ship outfitted and waiting for Covid patients but it was left unused. I only had my hospital to compare, and it was entirely different. No wonder people were dying, but it was a dramatic feed on the news cycle.

I was grateful that with the medical care my family was getting, we were indeed blessed. I was looking forward to resuming our Sibling Sundays and planning our next RV trip, the jaunts to the University of California San Francisco to visit my doctors with my sister, then on to lunch in Sausalito…and, of course, shopping… we both loved to shop! I had just gotten my Macy's Red Card and Sandy was a pro at getting the best deals. She had talked me into it before we left for Florida and I was looking forward to my "training sessions."

I had been home six days when Sam crept down the hallway. It was very early in the morning, but I was already sitting in my chair. Even behind the mask, I thought there was something different about his approach. He knelt outside my doorway and quietly told me that my sister Sandy had passed away that morning.

I began to cry out, but my breath caught. I gasped for air. The anguish I felt at that moment is indescribable. Never in my life have I felt such deep sorrow. At first, I thought it was a hallucination, then I reasoned it really didn't happen. I was so distraught. Sam couldn't hold me or comfort me physically due to the quarantine rules. I did not know if I could infect him and Christian. I had prayed daily. My friends were praying. She was on prayer chains, and yet, she did not survive.

Please God, not my sister. My grief was over-whelming. My thoughts turned to Jim and their children and grandchildren. Her first great-grandchild had been born in February. Her grandson was getting married in June to a girl my sister adored. I understood her excitement over their wedding.

Oh, please God, make this nightmare go away. I will never forget how Sam looked when he told me my sister had lost her battle with Covid. My breath caught again and again. The pain was so deep and seemed to go on forever. It must be a dream or one of my hallu-cinations. Yes, that is it. Sam didn't really say she was dead. It cannot be true.

God wouldn't bring us so close and then yank her away like that. She'd become my best friend, my confi-dant. I didn't have the chance to see her, talk with her, or say goodbye. How could this be happening?

Here I was, alone in my room. No hugs of comfort allowed. I had no idea if I was Covid free, or if I could give it to my husband or grandson. I needed comfort. I needed words of loving-kindness. My pain was so for-eign to me. I had lost both parents, but nothing prepared me for this loss.

I couldn't call anyone as my voice was not recov-ered from being on the ventilator and talking made breathing difficult.

Meanwhile, Kate was allowed in the hospital room with Rick to hold his hand and deliver the news. Glen was still receiving oxygen therapy so his family chose not to tell him. It was dreadfully painful when he phoned that morning to ask if I had any news on our siblings, and I was forced to lie. Instead of sharing our grief together, I had to pretend all was right with the world.

Reality is cruel. Being isolated compounds the cruelty. Guilt becomes my constant companion. Why did I survive? Did I give my siblings Covid? Why did my sister's kidneys fail? Why, why, why?! Life would never return to normal.

I began to look forward with great anticipation to my showers. Even though I wore my oxygen in the shower, the activity of showering, toweling off, and sometimes drying my hair made me so exhausted, I had to take a nap. Which meant my feelings of loss could not invade my world. I could rest for at least a brief time.

The ensuing days were filled with the routine of recovery. I had been given a second chance. My sister's passing made me all the more determined to recover fully. I had to be fit and healthy in case I was needed to help with my brother-in-law Jim or my brother Glen.

My skin was spotted with ugly red marks resembling the eraser end of a #2 pencil, and it was so dry it peeled off. I applied creams every few hours and exercised my legs so I could eventually stand and walk without the aid of a walker. I knew I could not change what happened. I was numb at times.

Exercises consisted of standing up from a seated position and repeating it ten times, leg lifts, and marching around with my walker. Exciting stuff.

I was fortunate enough to have two windows in my bedroom. One faced the porch in front of our home. I was able to see the delivery of flowers and food. I could wave to the generous providers. I looked forward to receiving the mail and the wonderful cards of encouragement. I have kept each and every one.

Propped up on my adjustable bed, I was able to watch the birds enjoying the spring and the squirrels scampering along the three-foot-high solid rock wall. Occasionally, one of the neighborhood peacocks would put on a colorful performance and drape its splendid plumes before me.

Thus, were my days. In between, my thoughts would return to my sister. Sandy had never been a concert-goer, but when Garth Brooks was coming to Sacramento, she was all in. We grabbed our cowgirl hats, threw on jeans and boots, and had Sam "limo" us to the arena. We had great seats and great seatmates. We were not the best singers in the group but were possibly among the loudest.

I never once gave thought to my life without her sharing in all the shenanigans. We had recently decided it was time to restart the tradition of going to Lake Tahoe for three days for the women in our families. We would go on the first weekend in October to celebrate my mom's birthday. We rented a large house on the beach at Zephyr Cove. Those days, which we called the

Farlee Follies, were never-ending laughs with a bit of gambling thrown in.

Finally, my fourteen-day quarantine was ending. I could go outside for a walk. I rose early in anticipation. I got dressed and ready. When you consider I had to take an oxygen canister, a walker, and my beloved Bernese, this was no simple undertaking.

By the time I was geared up and Sam and Christian had helped me to the end of the driveway, I could go no further. I was crushed. I was out of breath even with the aid of two liters of supplemental oxygen and a walker. Disappointment doesn't begin to describe what I considered a defeat. I had already cried every day since my sister's passing. Now, this day was even more tearful. Recovery was going to be work. My hopes of kayaking by August were dimming.

I was determined to be free of using supplemental oxygen AND going kayaking, my favorite activity. I rose every morning and walked further and further by doing the same distance for three or four days, then going a few feet further, until I reached my goal of one mile. My next goal was to see how far I could walk without supplemental oxygen.

I was pretty much left on my own to exercise and recover. Walking by myself was a necessity. I found walking with others and talking caused my oxygen levels to lower, which is quite detrimental for breathing!

I began my devotional time and talking to God about my thoughts and feelings. I was angry my sister had been taken from me. I was angry there could be no services, no celebration of life, no gathering of friends and family. The only choice was cremation. Nowhere for me to go to sit quietly and speak to her. I was not alone. Imagine how many others across the country were denied this part of the grieving process.

I was further angered by the fact that two high-profile political funerals were held with hundreds in attendance, but they were not considered "super-spreaders." Such hypocrisy at a time of national crisis.

Sam cooked, cleaned, and sanitized daily. Desperate Dinners became his favorite website. The housework, and taking care of Christian, and I gave him little rest.

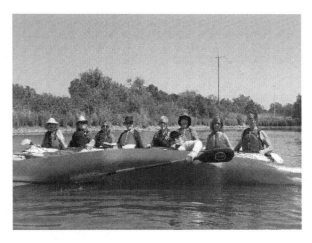

Enter my friend Karen and some of the BV Girls, my old schoolmates, and kayaking buddies. She organized a food train that fed us for two months. These were complete meals, often including dessert, and, occasionally, gifts for Christian. We had our first taste of Matzo Ball soup and others' special family recipes. It was a tremendous help as I was very weak. In addition, being hooked up to supplemental oxygen 24/7 meant I could not go near my gas range.

After two months, I was walking from my drive to the neighbors on my right and then back to my neighbors on the left. Yay me! The nap afterward was my reward.

Honk! Honk! What was this? During my recovery, my wonderful friend Karen organized a group who piled into their cars with painted signs, balloons, and decorations, and rolled past my home. My "honking hug parade" had begun. A few parked and stood on my walkway with signs of love and support. What an incredible feeling. I was so touched tears of happiness began to flow slowly down my cheeks.

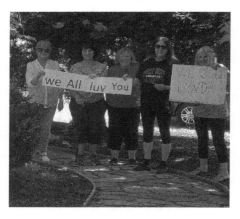

Meanwhile, Glen had been released from the hospital with a spirometer, a simple device to improve his lung capacity, as well as an oxygen tank with a very long cord. He had also been diagnosed with diabetes. The heavy use of certain medications to fight Covid had side effects. Diabetes was just one of them.

Glen's daughter came to check on him and care for him every single day. It was the best medicine he could have asked for. She was not prepared for how weak he was and how much care he needed right after his discharge. About two months after his discharge, he was no longer dependent on oxygen and he was out and about, grocery shopping, cooking, and, of course, going to doctor's appointments.

Rick was released to a convalescent hospital about two weeks after I had been released. He was extremely weak. Still, Kate was excited by the progress. He was to be there for two weeks, so she ordered an adjustable bed to be delivered before he came home. Surprise. After only a few days he was ready to come home. Like me, all those weeks in the hospital were enough. Of course, he arrived home before the new bed could be delivered.

His daughter, Katie, has her doctorate in physical therapy. She came four to five times a week and made sure he did his exercises. He was sent home with supplemental oxygen since he lives in a higher elevation but seldom had a need for it. His recovery was slow but steady.

The surgeon who had inserted his "peg" tube did not want him to come to the surgery center to have the tube removed, so his hospital doctor came to his home and removed it for him. Again, an amazingly compassionate medical professional continuing to be supportive.

As the days passed, my anxiety over recovery increased. I missed my sister. I missed seeing my brothers. About six weeks after my release from the hospital was Rick's birthday. I called him up and invited myself to his house. It would be my first outing, even if I would have to drag a portable oxygen tank down the steps to his patio.

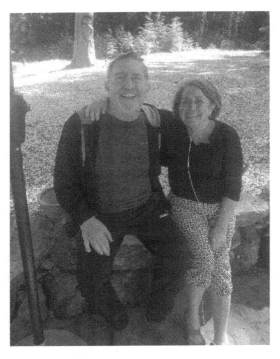

We all LOVE chocolate, so I purchased a double chocolate cake, ice cream, and goodies, and away we went. Tears formed upon seeing each other. It was an emotional time.

Later his daughter Katie, my former sister-in-law, Karen, and my adorable and charming nieces joined us for the celebration. Relaxing by the stone fire pit made life seem a bit more normal.

My first appointment with my pulmonary specialist was an eye-opener. Being one who has always envisioned a positive outcome of any occasion and planned accordingly, my disappointment was real.

I thought having COPD was an ugly diagnosis I had received years ago and did not want. I feel I sort of won that one. Now I was being diagnosed with a new lung disease; Covid Lung, of which there is little history or knowledge for progression or outcomes. I was a rare survivor, and it was still early on in the pandemic. My doctor gave me little encouragement that I would not be required to use supplemental oxygen for the rest of my life. As I envisioned a life tethered to a breathing apparatus, no kayaking, cooking, or regular activities, I silently thought, NOT AN OPTION!

I was anxious to get started on pulmonary therapy just to prove him wrong. But when I asked when I could start, the apologetic look on his face warned me I would not like his answer. There was such little known about this virus that the fear of cross-contamination of equipment meant recovering Covid patients, of which there were not yet many, could not attend pulmonary therapy classes until the medical profession had a clearer understanding of how to keep everyone safe.

I had expected to be able to kayak by August 2020. This news further dashed those hopes and expectations. Well, I had plans for a full return to normal life no matter what, so I got on Amazon and ordered a spirometer, as well as an oximeter to measure my oxygen levels and pulse rates. I also ordered a backpack to carry my portable oxygen and I geared up to defeat the effects of Covid.

I had survived. I was walking a mile a day with the help of oxygen. I felt I should be able to recover fairly quickly. The worst was over, right? Those were my assumptions. And those around me supported and encouraged my thoughts as well.

I have always looked for the "lesson" that can be learned from adversity, rather than be "woe is me." My grandmother was a great example of who I didn't want to be. I have never known an unhappier person. When I went to Ellis Island and looked her up, there it was— Anna "Woe is Me" Abegglen on the immigration registry.

I was no stranger to fighting my way through disease. Years ago, I had been hospitalized with what turned out to be a major Lupus flare-up. It was my first blood gas test and a diagnosis of lifelong debilitation. Nope...not doing it. Not living my life like that. I was so weak I could not get out of bed. When I finally made it out of bed, I had to crawl to the bathroom. I had a two-story home, but that couldn't stop me. I was determined to crawl down the stairs, even though I had to nap on the couch before going back up.

At that time, my neighbor and good friend, Gail, was recovering from esophageal cancer surgery. We made a pact to get stronger together. One day we agreed to go out our respective front doors and see each other and wave, then go back into our homes. We repeated this, and then made it to our mailboxes, then around the cul-de-sac. Walking the neighborhood was next. It took many months, but finally, we were walking several miles. Yay, us!

I also researched diets and only took one medication with an occasional series of prednisone. I adapted to a new normal. I had another major disease which is treated through the University of San Francisco Medical Center and once again, adapted to a new normal…so Covid was not to be any different.

Obviously, it is going to be more of a challenge as no historical data or record of recovery outcomes has been established. It will be up to me to find and refine diets, exercises, lung expansion, and anything else related to this disease. The fact that so little is known, and the symptoms and severity are not yet predictable, adds to the challenge.

As the summer progressed, I got up, dressed, strapped on my oxygen, and walked. One day I noticed a painted rock resting on a landscape stone in my front yard. It had a rainbow above a white fluffy cloud and the word HOPE. I knew it had to be one of my neighbors. Sure enough, my neighbor Michelle and her niece had left this note of encouragement. As the weeks passed, there were more rocks. A flamingo with One Step at a Time, a frog, a heart saying Stay Strong, another Bee Happy, and Bear Hugs with a Panda face. Another neighbor left an American Flag rock for the 4th of July. Such encouragement. Who wouldn't keep walking?

I was meeting my goals. I no longer needed 24/7 oxygen, especially at night. Finally, after five months, I could walk without supplemental oxygen.

Summers in the Sacramento Valley can be brutal

and this summer was no exception. In July and early August, the heatwave came. Temperatures above 105 degrees each day with no delta breeze coming in at night to cool things off. Next came the fires. Days when the sun was hidden by layers of smoke. You could see ash in the air and settling on outdoor furniture. The air quality was horrific; too bad to walk outside. The gyms and malls were closed because of Covid, eliminating my chance for indoor walking except within my home. This was a huge setback in my progress.

Our anniversary was in September so I excitedly made reservations at what has been our favorite beach-side escape for over thirty years. I couldn't wait to get out of the heat and smoke of the valley. We would be steps from the beach and the sound of the surf at Todd's Point. SURPRISE! It was the eeriest drive ever. Midway through the four-hour drive, around noon, the sky turned dark and we had to turn on our headlights.

It was like being in the twilight zone. No sun, no sky, just darkness. There would be no escape. Fallen ash was everywhere, including our balcony. We had "Helen Keller" waves. We could hear them but could not see them. No magical sunsets. Oh well, plenty of time for indoor activities. After all, it was our anniversary.

It was October before the air cleared. My recovery seemed to stall so I was excited to take the pulmonary function test that would allow me to go to high elevations and fly. As long as I breathed "consciously," I passed.

I booked a flight to surprise my friend Louise in

Laguna Niguel for her birthday in late October. My first "test." She and I had taken a trip to France and Barcelona two years earlier and developed a deep appreciation for European pastries and breads. Our quest since has been to find something similar here. Our first stop was a hidden gem in Laguna Hills called Chaupin Bakery—a bit of heavenly delights. I'm sure I gained a few pounds just by breathing in the aromas. We walked around Dana Point for our exercise, and as long as I took my supplemental oxygen along everything went well.

Upon my return, Sam and I immediately made plans to visit North Star near Lake Tahoe, Christian's favorite place. He has his own bedroom en-suite which makes him think he is "King." We were not there more than a few hours when my oxygen levels dropped. I had only been using my personal oxygenator, which requires conscious breathing. Still, at an altitude of around 6,500 feet, I couldn't get enough oxygen to keep my levels up. And I could not use the portable oxygen while sleeping as it is not a continuous flow delivery machine. Never even considered that. Believe me, I tried. We had originally planned on being there five nights but packed up after only two.

During my hospital stay, I had strained my shoulder muscles from pulling myself up in bed, so it was off to physical therapy in the fall also. Recovery and healing are such a process: lungs, muscles, neurological "surprises."

In August, my dear cousin who lives near Phoenix called. Her beloved husband had been hospitalized with

Covid. They had followed all the protocols. Isolated and only left home twice a month for groceries and necessities, yet, here they were. Although she could not be with him, he was able to facetime and communicate. He seemed to be doing pretty well, and then they placed him on the ventilator. Sadly, he passed away.

She wasn't the only one. I learned that several of my children, as well as friends, had also contracted Covid but recovered. My new grandson Rico's grandfather had been hospitalized and was on the ventilator for weeks. He was critically ill and then, one day, he opened his eyes, gradually got better, and was able to leave the hospital. He too had a long recovery.

Chapter 8 – Endings and Beginnings

While my family attempted to vacation in the early fall, the unthinkable happened. My brother-in-law, Jim, had been rushed to the hospital. Kidney failure. After his hospitalization, he was transferred to a convalescent hospital. He was home briefly, then returned to the hospital. It was the week before Thanksgiving when we learned he would not be recovering and had a short time to live. Again, another stressful, anguish-filled time for the family. Jim joined Sandy in death two days after Thanksgiving.

That same week my brother Glen was diagnosed with cancer. The holiday season was about to begin, yet heavy hearts hung abundantly. There was no family Christmas in 2020. Will there be one in 2021. Perhaps.

Now that only Glen, Rick, and I remain, mortality has become a dreaded reality. This past year has been one not only of reflection but stark truth. There has to be a reason I say to myself. I talk with God, and yet, I don't receive an answer. Why is He silent?

Being upbeat and positive by nature I do not recognize the symptoms of depression setting in. I am feeling overwhelmed, anxious. Sleep is elusive. I am exhausted most days but only "old people" take naps. I fight to stay awake.

Who am I kidding? I got Covid at age 72. I came close to death. My body went through an enormous amount of stress. My sister, as well as her husband, passed away. I came close to losing my baby brother as well. I did not have the energy to decorate my home for Christmas or entertain. The holidays are over. It is now 2021. I pray with gratitude in my heart, yet I do not feel the peace I am seeking.

Isolation is making people vulnerable to physical, mental, and emotional challenges. Prisoners are placed in isolation as a severe form of punishment. Now an entire world is being punished and held hostage to a mysterious virus.

I finally ask my doctor about my anxiety. He reviewed my year, looked at me, and said, "Just one of the events you have experienced this past year could cause stress and anxiety." He suggested a mild medication to help me relax.

This was not something with which I was comfortable. What if I became addicted? Do I have to take the pill forever? I realized I was afraid to admit I was overwhelmed with grief, guilt, and loneliness. I also had to admit I was powerless. For a Type-A driver personality, that is a hard pill to swallow. I had been wearing my, "I am okay, positive mask."

This admission of being powerless actually turned

out to be empowering. Crazy, I know, but it relieved me of so many negative thoughts that had been occupying my mind for these past months. Guilt had been my shadow, wondering if I was the source of Covid in my family, followed closely by grief and loneliness.

I came to understand the frustrating angry and often fearful social media posts. Our nation had been relentlessly pummeled with negative, discouraging, fear-filled opinions for an entire year. Kindness and mutual respect had been replaced by vitriolic rhetoric on both sides of the political divide. Moral credibility had all but disappeared.

I reached out once again to the hospital's Pulmonary Therapy program. They had promised Covid compliant classes since September, but nothing came of it. I was no longer going to accept their excuses. I called the director and was quite direct with my feelings of disappointment and anger. Why were Covid patients denied the opportunity to get the best chance of full recovery? Had not nine months been long enough for them to resolve the contamination issue? Penalizing survivors was not fair.

I then asked if she had ever been discriminated against or had people fearful of breathing the same air? Having people stay away from you and treat you like a leper? Harsh I know but within one week I was in class, learning how to breathe. Almost nine months after my release from the hospital. Fear of this virus by some in the medical profession had detoured my recovery long enough. I had regained my sense of hope through the support of family and friends. They EXPECTED me to recover fully, although they all admit to days of despair and fear. I was not going to disappoint.

I had been given the opportunity to live, against the odds. I could not let this opportunity be wasted. I have an obligation to do well. To get better. To make life count, not only for me but for everyone I encounter. My friends and family who had cried, prayed, and supported Sam and Christian through the dark days deserved to have me not only recover but rediscover the true meaning of love and friendship.

Chapter 9 – We Are All Essential

Essential is such an interesting term: essential workers, essential services. It seems the government chose winners and losers when they coined the phrase. Depending on who you talk to, and the timing, whether you are an essential winner or loser changes. Essential workers like doctors and nurses with too little knowledge about Covid and too few supplies and beds could be considered losers while they were attending non-stop to infected patients. But they became winners when the vaccine was finally available, being the first in line to get it.

I chose to adopt the term essential as part of my recovery, but with a different interpretation. Our family dynamics have changed forever, however, my brothers and I remain close.

I determined them to be ESSENTIAL.

I finally understand the limitations of time. There truly are only twenty-four hours in a day, and those hours are a precious gift that will never come again.

There is no guarantee I will have a tomorrow. I came to see spending time with "essential" family and friends must be a priority. Taking care of my health is essential. Laughing is essential.

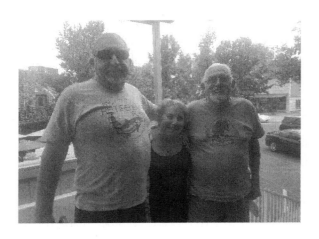

All of this means that in order to live the best version of what life I have left, I need to be the best wife, mother, sister, friend, cousin, etc. I can be. But to be the best, I know I can only invest deeply in a few relationships. I must be intentional. I have six children, two sons-in-law, two daughters-in-law, fifteen grandchildren, three great-grandchildren, and one on the way. I want to know the hopes, dreams, and aspirations of all my children and grandchildren. What is important to them? Who are their heroes or do they have one? What are they passionate about? Can I join in the activity or at least learn about it and support it? I want them to know the real me. The same is true for my close friends.

This does not mean I eliminate all others from my

life. It means I can still have relationships with many people, but there are only a finite number of people I can deeply invest time in, as that takes a great amount of intent and dedication.

I had always been a positive, outgoing person but in the past few years, I became overwhelmed with what I thought I needed to do and lost that crazy spark for life my friends had come to know.

I saw things not as they are, but as I would like them to be. I have caused anger, pain, joy, and happiness but my desire now is for more closeness, intimacy, and a whole lot of laughter.

Covid is an equal opportunity virus. Anyone, young, old, sick, healthy, thin, fat, can get it. Although for most, it is generally not that serious, I was blessed to have survived. I see this as a second chance to be a better wife, mother, Oma, Great-Grandma, neighbor, friend, human.

I had taken for granted that I would always have my sister, my brothers, family, neighbors, and friends. Funny how we so easily take for granted everyday life.

I began to dream, hope, and live with a renewed enthusiasm. I began to limit my social media exposure. I found there were many people who I did not know on my Facebook pages. How did that happen? A few minutes "peek" easily becomes wasted hours in your day if you are not watchful.

Personal phone calls and personal messages became my goal. Walking every day and seeking out those who were not afraid of me increased my socialization exposure.

I began seeking ways to connect with people. Real connections. I had never been good at that. I had used a "different" personality, different style of dress, as well as speech, depending on the situation. Always assessing what would be the appropriate attire, what expectations and images were applicable. Not a recipe for transparency. I am finding my voice and appreciating with sincere gratitude the people who have been with me pre-Covid, as well as through this difficult year. They continue to send me cards and call me, sharing life with me as I face the uncertainty of what Covid has done and the uncertainty of future discoveries about the effects of this virus.

I have wonderful memories. Mother's Day brunch that Todd and his family brought over and shared on our patio six weeks after my hospital release. Celebrating my brother Rick's birthday. Enjoying the discovery of peacock feathers on my walks. The best Christmas in so very long.

A neighbor I have never actually met dropped by with a plate of homemade cookies. My daughter hand-painted a family tree. My son and daughter-in-law presented me with a book of personal memories my grandchildren wrote about me. My grandson and his precious wife presented me with an "Angel on my Shoulder" pin; my sister's birth month as the main stone.

Recently one of my neighbors stopped by with a bag of fresh lemons from her tree and a mocha from Starbucks. Catching up and getting to know her better made my day. I had not slept well and had just literally crawled out of bed. The old me would have been so embarrassed and uncomfortable. The visit would have been stilted, uncomfortable, and brief. But I invited her in and we relaxed and chatted for an hour and a half. And I got a promise of more lemons to boot. My passion is cooking and using lemons is not a problem. I love lemon anything!

Being an encourager by nature, I began reaching out to others. Taking the focus off of me, and sharing the lives of those who choose to be a part of my journey is my "new" life.

Sam and I have plans to travel with Christian and share the history and the beauty of our country while reconnecting with those we know in other states.

I no longer focus on how I would be perceived or how I should dress "appropriately" for events. The obsession with my image no longer dominates. I used to even determine in my mind how these events would unfold. You guessed it. Not good.

My image is no longer central in my thoughts. My hair is a throw-back to hippy days; wild, wavy curls. Can you say low maintenance? My style of dress? Whatever is comfortable at the time.

I have found my voice. Finally. Although I am evolving and discovering new things about myself and those around me, I highly recommend recognizing each day as a gift. Unwrap it with wonder and delight. Be a "gift" to those you encounter. But mostly be kind and loving to yourself.

TRUST in something greater than yourself. It will be different for everyone. For me, it means strengthening my relationship with Jesus Christ. Recently I heard a description of many Christians' prayer life. It resembles an Amazon shopping cart. You select what you want God to do, add it to the cart. Push order and set the delivery date for the prayer to be answered. I do not want to be that person.

Daily gratitude, hope, and a renewed spirit to embrace and enjoy life, no matter what happens along the way is my goal.

I invite all of you to join me by taking your own personal journey of discovery, and perhaps changing the world one day, one person at a time by watching less news, disengaging from social media, and reconnecting with family, neighbors, and friends. Mend fences where necessary, strengthen existing ties, and embrace true relationships.

> "This is the day the Lord hath made.
> Rejoice and be Glad in it"

About the Author

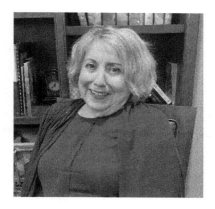

Lynda Armes was born in the Midwest but transplanted to Northern California at the age of two. She, along with her brothers and sister, grew up in idyllic times and established life-long relationships close to where they grew up.

Described as a Renaissance Woman by a long-time business colleague, Lynda is known for her fearless, positive attitude and a slant towards sometimes quirky shenanigans. Achieving the status of Real Estate Broker years back, along with extraordinary technological advances, gave her the independence to not only provide excellent service for her clients but the opportunity for travel, service to others, and to pursue her writing.

Her most memorable volunteer trips were serving in Sighisoara, Romania, which included an interesting five-hour 1930s train ride from Bucharest, as well as heart-wrenching experiences in the state institution orphanage. Romania was followed years later by a trip that included sweltering trips daily into the surrounding jungles of Monterio, Columbia, a few hours from Medellin with gang violence nearby. We took part in creative arts for children and provided encouragement and hope through enterprise and business development endeavors for both homeless and abused women.

Publishing this book has checked off her list an important life goal. The impetus for which was a life-altering experience. Her journey through Covid-19 was shared globally and touched millions of lives.

She currently resides with her husband, Samuel, ten-year-old grandson, Christian, and her beloved Bernese Mountain Dog Bernie, affectionately known as "The Million Dollar Dog," and universally loved by all who know him.

Her passion for helping the underserved, reading, writing, traveling, and kayaking are among her favorite things to do...surrounded by family and friends.

Lynda would love to start a conversation. If you have questions or would like to share a personal story, you may reach her at

LyndaArmes1@gmail.com

Acknowledgments

Kelli Robson, lovingly known as Nurse Kelli to close family and friends. She had the unenviable job of keeping everyone informed all the while knowing more than she could share at times.

Sutter Hospital Roseville ICU, Critical Care Covid Unit for their dedication in fighting this disease from the beginning.

Claire Lack Stevens, Karen Ramirez, and my amazing BV Girls for their unending encouragement and support.

My incredible neighbor Michelle Cemo and her niece for painting my "walk rocks."

All those who prayed, my neighbors who delivered food, gifts for Christian, and encouragement for Sam.

Kelly Resendez, who, through her Mastermind sessions, prayer support in the business community, and her book, *Big Voices,* gave me the courage to finally accomplish my biggest, oldest goal in life; to author a book.

Caren Cantrell, my editor. This book would have remained an unfulfilled dream of mine if it were not for her guidance, patience, and belief.

Kate Newman Farlee for capturing the perfect photos for my book cover.

Made in the USA
Columbia, SC
03 July 2021

41344269R00063